Sports and Traumatology

Series Editor
Philippe Landreau
Doha, Qatar

As more and more people are getting involved in sports, even the elderly, sports traumatology has become a recognized medical specialty. In sports exercises, every joint and every anatomical region can become the location of a traumatic injury: an acute trauma, a series of repeated microtraumas or even an overuse pathology. Different sports activities may produce different and specific traumas in the same anatomical region.The aim of the book series 'Sports and Traumatology' is to present in each book a description of the state of the art on treating the broad range of lesions and the mechanisms in sports activities that cause them. Sports physicians, surgeons, rehabilitation specialists and physiotherapists will find books that address their daily clinical and therapeutic concerns.

More information about this series at http://www.springer.com/series/8671

Gian Nicola Bisciotti • Piero Volpi
Editors

The Lower Limb Tendinopathies

Etiology, Biology and Treatment

Springer

Editors
Gian Nicola Bisciotti
Qatar Orthopaedic and
Sport Medicine Hospital
Doha
Qatar

Piero Volpi
Medical Departement FC. Internazional
Istituto Clinico Humanitas Milano(Italy)
Milan
Italy

ISSN 2105-0759 ISSN 2105-0538 (electronic)
Sports and Traumatology
ISBN 978-3-319-33232-1 ISBN 978-3-319-33234-5 (eBook)
DOI 10.1007/978-3-319-33234-5

Library of Congress Control Number: 2016951460

Printed on acid-free paper

This Springer imprint is published by Springer Nature
The registered company is Springer International Publishing AG Switzerland

Contents

Chapter 1
Tendonitis, Tendinosis, or Tendinopathy?

Gian Nicola Bisciotti and Piero Volpi

Abstract The term tendinopathy does not seem more suited to describe the processes that the tendon undergoes during its rearrangement in the case of its biological and structural distress. In effect, the inflammatory process would seem to be absent, or in any case very limited, from a temporal point of view, while it would seem to prevail the biological degeneration process. For this reason, it would seem preferable to use the term "tendinopathy." In effect, this term would describe much better the profound processes of biological and structural rearrangement that the tendon suffers. However, one cannot ignore the fact that often inflammatory and degenerative processes can coexist.

1.1 Introduction

Historically the term "tendonitis" was used to describe chronic painful symptoms on a tendon with overt algic symptoms, a concept which implied the existence of an inflamed state as a primary disease process. However, in spite of this definition, the fact that normal anti-inflammatory therapies became more evident showed very limited effect on the aforementioned tendonitis [1, 2]; simultaneously to this statement, the results of the first studies of histology appeared in literature, which showed the presence, in such clinical pictures, of a degenerative process which was coexistent with that of inflammation. All of this put seriously into doubt the concept of

G.N. Bisciotti (✉)
Qatar Orthopaedic and Sports Medicine Hospital, FIFA Center of Excellence, Doha, P.O. Box 29222, Qatar
e-mail: bisciotti@libero.it

P. Volpi
Humanitas Clinical Institute, IRCCS, Rozzano, Milan, Italy
FC Internazionale Medical staff, Milan, Italy

G.N. Bisciotti, P. Volpi (eds.), *The Lower Limb Tendinopathies*, Sports and Traumatology, DOI 10.1007/978-3-319-33234-5_1

centrality of the same inflammation process of disease on the tendon tissue [3, 4]. Ever since then the term tendonitis was progressively abandoned, to be substituted by a more generic term, that of "tendinopathy."

1.2 The Histological Aspect of the Tendon Affected by Tendinopathy

From a point of view of structural framework, in the healthy tendon, the fibers are laid in a parallel way and are strongly linked to one another. On the other hand, in the injured tendon, the fibers show a clear increase of their wavy aspect and a marked structural separation, thus showing a clear loss of their normal structure. In the tendinopathic tendon – or one which has maintained its continual structure, in spite of the development of disease – we can observe an increase of the wavy aspect of the fiber which is less accentuated in regard to that of the injured one. The nuclei of the tenocytes of the affected tendon by tendinopathy generally appear flat and tapered and, sometimes, distributed in line. In the case of severe tendinopathy, the tenocytes assume an aspect similar to chondrocytes. In the injured tendon, the tenocytes appear smaller and the nuclei are rounded. In some cases, the injured tendons show anarchic vascularization, often linked with the degenerative process; this neovascularization runs parallel to the collagen fibers. We may also observe an increase in glycosaminoglycans (GAG) which could influence the structure of the fibro and their organization, inducing a reparative response which can contemplate even a neovascularization process [5]. Histologically the changes of degenerative character are classified as:

(i) Hypoxic
(ii) Hyaline
(iii) Mucoid and myxoid

Furthermore, to this situation is often associated – above all in some specific tendon areas, for example, the rotator cuff – a lipid degeneration.

1.3 The Coexistence of Degenerative and Inflammatory Changes

Many authors agree on the fact that phenomena such as inflammation and degeneration may rarely be shown in an isolated way and which instead, more often, coexist in adjacent areas of the observed anatomic sample [2, 6–8]. Generally, in fact, macroscopic changes, at an intra-tendon level, in the case of tendinopathy, may be described as the formation of a scarcely marked area inside which we can identify a focal loss of the tendon structure. The tendon portion affected by tendinopathy loses its translucid aspect, and it appears grayish and amorphous. The tendon appears much thicker, in a fusiform and nodular way, and inside we may sometimes observe calcification, fiber calcification, and bone metaplasia. The different portions of the degenerated tendon area show an ample variety regarding cellular density; in fact in some areas, we may observe an increase of the contextual cellular density and a high rate of metabolic activity. On the other hand, we may observe only a few pyknotic[1] cells in certain areas, or we may compare their total absence. Some changes in disease are often observed even in the tendon matrix, where we can frequently observe contextual mucoid material by a separation of the collagen fibers. The collagen fibers usually show irregularity, a difference and an increase in their crimping, as well as a loss of visibility in the transversal band. The degenerated fibers may be replaced by calcification areas or by infiltrated lipids, which give origin to the tendolipomatosis phenomena. A clear increase may be noted in the type III collagen which is poor, with respect to type I collagen, concerning the number of cross-links between and inside the tropocollagen units [9]. In spite of the evidence of such degenerative alterations, in the tendon tissue affected by tendinopathy, their clinical relevance is still not clear. Degenerative hypoxia, mucoid degeneration, calcification, and tendolipomatosis all represent phenomena which, either singularly or together, are visible in a high percentage of tendons in healthy and asymptomatic individuals at the age of 35 years and over [5, 10].

In the case of tendinopathy, we may observe frequent changes in the peritendinous structure, which appear more often in tendons showing a synovial sheath – i.e., posterior tibia, peroneal, and flexors and extensors of the wrist and of the fingers [11, 12]. In the acute phase of tendinopathy, in the histological examination, we may frequently see the presence of fibrinous exudates, followed by a second phase characterized by a diffused proliferation of fibroblasts. Following a macroscopic observation, the peritendinous tissue appears thick, and phenomena of adhesion are often visible between the tendon and paratenon [2]. During a chronic phase, the main cells of the paratenon are fibroblasts and myofibroblasts. Regarding the myofibroblasts, it is interesting to note that during the remodeling process, the fibroblasts assume their own characteristics, both from a morphological and biochemical point of view of the contractile cells. For this reason they are defined as myofibroblasts. The myofibroblasts possess a modest amount of actin inside their cytoplasm and thus have a certain contractile capacity. Due to these characteristics, the myofibroblasts may induce and maintain, in time, a lengthened state of contraction in a frame of peritendon adhesion, causing, at the same time, a state of vascular constriction perturbing intra-tendon circulation, which then probably starts up a reactive process of vascular proliferation. For some authors, peritendinitis is a process of inflammatory nature [2].

In an animal model – specifically the rabbit – damage provoked to the tendon tissue causes an infiltration of inflammatory cells which becomes evident at a distance of 6 h; on the other hand, when damage to the tendon tissue is provoked by

[1] *Pyknosis: in cytology, the contraction of the cell nucleus (pyknotic core) or of all the protoplasm, which looks like a mass intensely colored without regular pattern. It is generally a degeneration sign.*

overuse, we may merely observe histological changes of degenerative type [13, 14]. Still in an animal model, this time equine, the superficial flexor tendons of the digits undergoing overload show a precocious phase of inflammatory type, followed by a phase of degenerative type [15, 16]. These experiments, even though out of date, induce us to consider the hypothesis that the inflammatory process may represent the precocious phase of the tendinopathic process, to which follows a second phase of degenerative type, even if we have to admit that the relationship between the two phenomena is to date still not clear. Further studies, still on an animal model, show the existence of damage of oxidative type and an increase of the apoptotic phenomena when tendon structure is put under chronic stress [17]. Studies executed on rabbits have proven that mastocytes adjacent to the neural structure release neuropeptides – in particular neuropeptide substances P (SP) and calcitonin gene-related peptide (CGRP) – as well as specific mediators (mast cell mediator) such as histamine, prostaglandin, and leukotrienes able to influence both the activity of the fibroblasts and the vascular permeability [18].

Studies carried out on man are obviously more pertinent than those on animals; however, we must consider the fact that almost all of the studies carried out on man are performed on symptomatic tendons representing undoubted limitation. In such a way, it is rarely possible to observe the first phase, asymptomatic, of tendinopathy. Therefore, the main studies carried out on man may be interpreted by considering such limitation of the experimental model. In studies done by Alfredson [4], the authors refer how the level of prostaglandins E2 (PGE2) is similar in the case of chronic tendinopathy as in the case of absolute biological and histological normality, excluding the presence of an inflammatory process in later phases of the tendinopathic process. Yang and colleagues are not of the same opinion [19], who, on the other hand, observe how the mechanical stress on the patellar tendon induces and increases the production of PGE2 on behalf of the fibroblasts. The PGE2, as well as representing a strong inhibitor of the synthesis of collagen type I [20–22], shows a marked catabolic effect to the damage of the tendon structure where inhibition of the collagen production is provoked [23]. Other experiments show us how the levels of lactate grow significantly in the diseased tendon, witnessing the fact that the majority of anaerobic mechanisms of the tendon affected by tendinopathy represents the answer to the insufficiency of oxygen to the tissue [24, 25]. This hypothesis is confirmed by the fact that hypoxia observed in the suffering tendons of degenerative phenomena induces the production of hypoxia-inducible factor which, in turn, provokes the expression of vascular endothelial growth factor (VEGF) [26, 27]. Apart from its angiogenic properties, the VEGF is able to provoke an upregulation of the expression of matrix metalloproteinase (MMP) which, in turn, increases the degradation of extracellular matrix (ECM) altering the mechanical properties of the tendon [28, 29, 30]. The neoangiogenesis is followed by a proliferation of the nervous terminals and by the production of algogenic substances which, together with a high level of glutamate, typically found in tendinopathy, are the responsible factors of the outbreak of algic symptoms [2]. All these mechanisms may lead to a situation of repeated microtraumas which may show in a tendon breakage.

1.4 Study Models of Tendinopathy

Studies of tendinopathy disease carried out on man, even though being, without doubt, of the most interest, meet difficult objectives. Human tissue obtained surgically, or by biopsy, generally come from subjects who have developed advanced disease, without taking into account difficult objective in finding healthy tendon samples to use as a control model. For this reason, to the end of deepening the knowledge of mechanisms which determine the outbreak of tendinopathy, model tendons are used which may be in vitro, ex vivo, or in vivo.

1.4.1 In Vitro Models

In literature we find some interesting studies, carried out in vitro, based on chronic reminders in the lengthening of the tendon. The chronic stretching of the tendon structures is, in fact, considered as one of the main risks of the development of tendinopathy. In studies in vitro of this type, in general, they undergo a stretching cycle of the tenocytes or of the fibroblasts, and the mechanic strain has the aim of observing the effects of cellular deformation of potential cellular mediators and molecules [31]. Some of the studies [32–34] have highlighted how the deformation of tenocytes and fibroblasts have determined an increase in the production of PGE2, cyclooxygenase-1 (COX-1), cyclooxygenase-2 (COX-2), cytosolic phospholipase A1 (cPLA1), secretory phospholipase A2,[2] and leukotrienes B4. Some authors [19] have underlined the importance of the role of interleukin-1β (IL-1β) in the inflammatory process in a human model in vitro made up of fibroblasts of the patellar tendon. The authors noticed that, when IL-1β was present, a lengthening cycle of the tendon fibers equal to 4 % was sufficient to cause a decrease in the expression of COX-2, of the MMP-1, and of the production of PGE2; on the contrary, a lengthening cycle equal to 8 % of the length of the fibers showed an increase of the expression MMP-1. So, the conclusions of the study were that moderate stretching showed an anti-inflammatory effect, whereas more accentuated stretching ended in a pro-inflammatory action. The advantages of the experiments in vitro in the studies of tendinopathy present the allowance of observation in a simple and quick way of a good number of cellular processes, for example, the synthesis of DNA, mitosis, the genic expression, and the cellular differentiation [32, 34–42]. As well as this undoubted advantage, during the experiments in vitro, cells may undergo lengthening in a similar way to that of what happens in an in vivo situation. This latter aspect carries particular importance, as a change in the mechanism of lengthening may involve a different type of cellular response [43]. However, we must note that during such type of experiment, we may see that the inconvenience that the lengthening

[2] *The phospholipase A2 are enzymes that have the task to separate the fatty acids from the oxidized phospholipids.*

imposed on the substratus is not completely transferred to the cell, becoming imprecise both in length of time and frequency [44]. In any case, the main limitation of in vitro studies is represented by the fact that the study of isolated cells in an environment avoided of cellular matrix (ECM) and neurovascular connections, limits the interpretation of the obtained results when we want to refer these latter in a situation of natural activation.

1.4.2 Ex Vivo Models

Ex vivo models provide, in tendinopathy, the possibility to observe and study the changes and answers to different stimuli by the entire tendon tissue and not only from a few isolated cells, as happens in in vitro models. These models allow interaction between the tendon cells and the ECM, which, remaining intact, is able to provide a biological environment so as to allow efficient control of the experimental conditions. The main methods of study applied in ex vivo models are cyclical loading, creep loading, and stress deprivation.

(i) *The cyclical loading*
Exactly as what happens in in vivo models, the cyclical loading (or cyclical stretching) in ex vivo models is carried out in order to observe the effects of a repeated chronical load on the tendon tissue which shows intact ECM. After about 24 h of cyclical loading, the tissue shows a decrease in value of the mechanic failure (ultimate failure strength), becoming significantly weaker from a structural point of view [45]. In such conditions, we also assist in an increase of cellular turnover and of the quantity of collagen and unmistakable signs of tissue degradation [46]. Devkota and colleagues [46] also noted how, when the tendon sample was put through cyclical loading, it was linked to the production of PGE2. Also the levels of MMP-1 would seem linked to the length and the frequency of the imposed load; low loading and low frequency would cause an inhibition of the expression MMP-1, whereas the application of high loads at high frequency would entail the complete inhibition of the expression [47]. Some authors recommend using, during cyclical loading, experiments done ex vivo on the tendon, tension superior to 5 % of the maximum supporting tension; it seems that for tension inferior to this level, we are not able to produce appreciable structural deformation [48, 49]. The ex vivo method doesn't entail the same complexity as the in vivo method. In fact, as in the in vitro method, during ex vivo experiments, the damage provoked by cyclical loading is not completely repaired; complete repair cannot come about both because of the absence of vascularization and the deficiency of molecules of the signaling systemic.

(ii) *Creep loading*
As well as a repetitive chronic load, a situation also reproduced during cyclical loading experiments, the tendon tissue may undergo structural damage also through the application of sustained and prolonged loading. This type of situation, during experiments in ex vivo, is reproduced by using the creep loading

method. In this environment, Wren and colleagues [49] studied the different intercurrents between the effects caused by cyclical loading and creep loading on the human Achilles tendon, observing in both cases a significant structural damage. So, both cyclical loading and creep loading represent two valid ways of investigation in the study of tendinopathy.

(iii) *Stress deprivation*
Studies on stress deprivation resolve the aim of observing changes induced by immobilization in the sample in question. In studies of this type – ex vivo, in vivo, and in vitro – the immobilization causes an increase in the expression MMP-1 mRNA, a factor which involves an expiry of the tensile characteristics of the tendon [47, 50, 51]. For such a reason, the experiments of stress deprivation represent a valid study model of tendinopathy. However, in this type of experiment, the tensile properties of the tendon are altered without which a simultaneous change in the diameter of the collagen fibers occurs. For this reason, experiments of stress deprivation are not adapt to the study of the role of collagen in the context of tendinopathy. A complete understanding of the processes which regulate the outbreak and the evolution of tendinopathy – even when referring to experiments in vitro and ex vivo, which represent an important model of understanding regarding a specific cellular answer – it cannot be exempt from the use of experiments in vivo. To this aim, numerous experimental models have been conceived and developed so as to induce specific answers, at a tendon level, before the application of interfering experiments of chemical and mechanic nature. The necessity of having more than one model available is dictated by the fact that each experimental model is able to represent only one aspect of disease in tendinopathy. A further important aspect to remember is represented by the fact that we are obliged to choose models coming from different animal species as well as knowing the gene sequence, because no animal model exists, which possesses tendons, with the same characteristics as that of humans [52]. There are advantages and disadvantages connected with the different methods of induction of tendinopathy based on chemical and mechanical induction. In the first case, for example, we receive an answer from the part of the tendon tissue of acute type, which does not represent changes induced from a chronic tendinopathy in the human tendon; on the other hand, however, chemical induction shows the advantage of being less laborious in comparison with a mechanical one and is able to induce consistent tendon damage.

1.4.3 In Vivo Chemical Induction Models

The in vivo chemical induction models (in vivo CIM) can be divided into four main categories. Depending on the different techniques used, we can in fact have:

(i) In vivo CIM injecting collagenase

(ii) In vivo CIM injecting cytokines
(iii) In vivo CIM injecting prostaglandins
(iv) In vivo CIM injecting fluoroquinolones

(i) In vivo CIM injecting collagenase
One of the chemical induction models of tendinopathy consists in injecting collagenase into the tendon undergoing experimentation. One of the first studies that used the injecting of collagenase in the tendon in order to induce a tendinopathic process was done by Foland and colleagues [53]. The animal model chosen was the horse, and the injecting of collagenase was performed in three different areas of the flexor digitorum superficialis tendon. The tendon reaction was the development of an injury in the injected area, with a consequent repair process implying the proliferation of collagen type III. Other similar experiments used the injecting of collagenase in the supraspinatus tendon in a mouse model [54], which induces a strong cellular increase, the destruction of the collagen organization, and the increase of vascular tissue. The effects of the injecting of collagenase were completely resolved and repaired only after a period of about 12 weeks [54] even though some authors have recently observed the persistence of the phenomena for a longer time, around 32 weeks [55]. In all these experiments, we may observe a substantial loss of an initial inflammatory process. However, other studies show that inflammation became evident after 15 days from the injecting of collagenase, and at a distance of 16 weeks, it was able to see a chondral metaplasia with ossification [56]. Even though through this type of experiment we may obtain many similar characteristics to those of a human tendon affected by tendinopathy – such as hypercellularity, loss of organization of the matrix, an increase in vascularization, and absence of an inflammatory process – we cannot ignore the fact that the injecting of bacterial collagenase in an animal model may present substantial differences from that of human collagenase and hence inducing likewise substantially different reactions [57, 58].

(ii) In vivo CIM injecting cytokines
Since tendinopathy may present, even in its precocious phase, a process of inflammatory type, followed by a second phase of degenerative type, the injecting of cytokines represents an experimental model whose aim is that of inducing an inflammatory reaction. Following this species-specific injecting of cytokines on a patellar tendon in a rabbit, Stone and colleagues [58] observed after 4 weeks an increase in cellularity which drifted toward normality only after about 16 weeks. However, the injecting of cytokines was able to provoke only slight and reversible structural damage, without damage to the matrix or the degradation of collagen. So, the injecting of cytokines would seem not to represent a trustworthy model in order to reproduce a tendinopathic process. In any case, since the injecting of cytokines is species specific, this method has the advantage of normalizing intraspecies differences.

(iii) In vivo CIM injecting prostaglandins
Since studies in vitro [31, 33] and in vivo [59] have shown that repetitive mechanical stress induces the production of prostaglandin, on behalf of fibroblasts in the

human tendon, the injecting of these may represent a valid study model of tendinopathies. In the first week of weekly administration of PGE1 on the Achilles tendon in mice, Sullo and colleagues [60] met a growing content of contextual water to an inflammatory process. In the third week, half of the treated tendons showed signs of fibrosis on the paratenon associated with adhesions and degeneration, whereas the other half showed evident signs of inflammation. In the fifth week, all the treated samples showed signs of fibrosis on the paratenon with adhesions and degeneration. The authors concluded that the repetitive injecting of PGE1 caused, at the beginning, an inflammatory process which then tended toward a degenerative state. Also, the repetitive injecting of PGE1 in the patellar tendon of the rabbit [61] caused an increase in cellularity, disorganization and degeneration of the collagen matrix, and a decrease in the diameter of the collagen fibrils. Furthermore, the processes of tendon degradation are directly linked to the dose of injected prostaglandin [61]. The injecting of prostaglandin on an animal model causes a sequence of phenomena similar to those in a human tendon, affected by tendinopathy which are hypercellularity, deformation and degeneration of the tendon structure, and dilution of the collagen fibrils. So, chemical induction models based on the injecting of prostaglandin show a valid model for study on tendinopathy in an animal model, even if further studies are necessary in order to obtain full comprehension of action mechanisms of the same prostaglandins.

(iv) In vivo CIM injecting fluoroquinolones

As is well known, the use of fluoroquinolones induces the onset of severe tendinopathy which may involve the complete breakage of the tendon [62–65]. Single administration of 300 or of 900 mg/kg of pefloxacin [7] (PFLX), or 900 mg/kg of ofloxacin (OFLX) in mice, causes an infiltration of pro-inflammatory cells of peritenon and of the Achilles tendon, contextual to a disorganization of collagen strips [66]. Following the administration of PFLX or OFLX, the fibroblasts presented a fragmentation of nuclei and showed signs of dead cells; such a picture tended to become less severe in the case of OFLX but not in the case of PFLX [64–66]. Some authors carried out analyses regarding the possible effects of different quinolones, observing a certain variability on the different tested products [67]. In each case, at least in mice, the more toxic fluoroquinolones, and thus causing more serious injuries on the Achilles tendon, would seem to be fleroxacin (FLX) and PFLX. Other fluoroquinolones show minor toxicity and cause tendon injuries only for doses between 300 and 900 mg/kg, whereas norfloxacin, ciprofloxacin, and tosufloxacin do not show adverse effects on tendon structure up until doses equal to 900 mg/kg [44]. Further studies show that the injuring mechanism on a tendon activated by the assumption of PFLX and FLX is represented by the inhibition of the synthesis of proteoglycans and by the induction of oxidative damage of collagen [67]. We may, therefore, conclude that, in mice, the administration of fluoroquinolones, in particular PFLX and FLX, induces the onset of tendinopathy with characteristics (injuries and edema) similar to those in the human tendinopathic tendon [68]. However, the injecting of fluoroquinolones in mice presents several important differences in comparison to that of the human. The major difference is made up of the fact that, in mice, the injecting of fluoroquinolones does not involve breakage of the tendon, as it does in man [65]. Furthermore, in man, even a low dose seems to involve much more serious effects on the structure of the tendon in comparison to that on mice. In the light of this data, we may affirm that the assumption of fluoroquinolones stimulates several specific reactions which induce the onset of severe tendinopathy in man (not showing in mice); this renders the mouse model less interesting in reproducing the effects of tendinopathy induced by the use of such pharmaceuticals.

1.4.4 In Vivo Mechanical Induction Models of Tendinopathy

The etiology of the overuse of tendinopathy is, in literature, largely shared [69–72]; for this reason an ample use of mechanical models of induction of tendinopathy has become widespread. Since the mechanical models are able to induce chronic tendinopathy, mainly taking advantage of an overuse mechanism, and not of acute tendinopathy as in chemical induction models, it appears clear that the application of a mechanical model is longer and more laborious. In literature, we find five categories of in vivo mechanical induction models of tendinopathy, of which we will briefly illustrate the main characteristics.

1.4.5 Mechanical Induction Models of Tendinopathy Based on Electrical Stimulus

Electrical exogenous stimulus of a muscle provokes a contraction which produces a flexo-extension movement which mechanically loads the relative tendon. Backmand and colleagues [13], by using electrostimulation (ES), managed to reproduce, on an animal model, tendinopathic processes with similar characteristics observed in man. The ES of the triceps muscle of a rabbit resulted in the tendon degeneration with neo-capillarization and the presence of pro-inflammatory cells. Also, Nakama and colleagues [73] and Asundi and colleagues [74] obtained similar results by electrostimulating the deep flexor of the digits of a rabbit. The ES thus represents a mechanical induction model of tendinopathy with satisfying reproducibility and relatively contained experimental timing. However, it is important to remember that some authors noted that ES may have different effects in different areas of the tendon undergoing experimentation [73, 74]. Furthermore, in some cases [75], an outbreak of tendinopathy was also seen in the contralateral tendon not undergoing ES, which could doubt the control conditions of the experimental protocol based on ES.

1.4.6 Mechanical Induction Model of Tendinopathy Based on Downhill Treadmill Running

Several experiments carried out on mice have proven to be like a downhill run – carried out with a 10 % incline, at the speed of 17 km/h, with the frequency of 1 h a day, 5 days a week, and for a variable number of weeks – done on a treadmill (downhill treadmill running, DTR) and induce severe structural changes on the tendon of the supraspinatus [76, 77]. The changes observed on the tendon included an increase in cellularity, a cell deformation, a nonalignment of the collagen fibers, and an increase of the cross-sectional area of the tendon: such structural alterations were evident for a period between 4 and 16 weeks. As well as these structural modifications, an increase of the genic expression of COX-2 was clear after 8 weeks, followed by its normality after about 16 weeks, whereas the VEGF values increase for the whole 16 weeks. This data proves the evidence both of the onset of inflammatory phenomena and of neoangiogenesis. Other experiments done with the DTR method evidenced an increase of the expression interleukin-18 (IL-18), interleukin-15 (IL-15), and interleukin-6 (IL-6) [78] and an increase in the expression of mediators in the process of apoptosis and of the levels of heat shock proteins (HSP).[3] In general, the DTR method may be considered a valid means of mechanical induction of tendinopathy. From a practical point of view, the method presents disadvantages connected to a long experimental period, necessary to induce the disease changes on the tendon, and undoubted difficulty in the training of guinea pigs. Furthermore, the DTR on mice would seem to affect only the supraspinatus tendon and not the Achilles one [79].

1.4.7 The Mechanical Induction Model of Tendinopathy Based on Uphill Treadmill Running

Since experiments carried out using the DTR method have not been able to show, in mice, tendinopathic induction on the Achilles tendon, some authors [80] introduced an experimental method based on uphill treadmill running (UTR). By using the UTR method, Glazebrook [80] obtained, on the Achilles tendon of mice, a disorganization of collagen fibers, contextual to a phenomena of neovascularity, and an increase in fibroblasts. So, the UTR method seems more adapt, in comparison with the DTR method, in inducing tendinopathy of the Achilles tendon in mice. The reason of this further efficiency in inducing tendinopathy of the Achilles tendon of the UTR method may be explained by the fact that uphill treadmill running requires a further eccentric activity of the complex muscle tendon involved [81], showing further tendon damage [82–84].

---

[3] *Heat shock proteins (HSP) are a class of functionally linked proteins, involved in folding and unfolding of other proteins.*

1.4.8 The Mechanical Induction Model of Tendinopathy Based on Fatigue

One of the most common etiological causes of tendinopathy is represented by a chronic overloading on the tendon able to alter the genic answer associated with the outbreak of the same tendinopathy. In other words, the fatigue phenomena may be in such conditions the *primum movens* of the outbreak in the tendinopathic process. Sun and colleagues [85], by inducing the fatigue phenomena through the application of cyclical loading on the patellar tendon of mice, of a magnitude between 1 and 35 N, with 1Hz frequency, managed to induce a series of microstructural damage together with an upregulation of MMP-13 and IL-1β. Using the same method, Fung and colleagues [86] showed the linking existence between the level of fatigue induced and the structural damage caused on the matrix and collagen fibers, as well as highlighting an increase in the expression of collagen of types III and V. The mechanical model based on the induction of fatigue, thus, was able to induce reproducible and controllable structural damage on the tendon of mice, showing, however, the limit of being able to induce such damage in an acute way or through an application of a single load, even if the application of the latter is reiterated in time, and not through chronic and intermittent mechanical stress, as is typical in man.

1.4.9 The Mechanical Induction Model of Tendinopathy Based on Disuse

Even though its effects are still not fully understood, several studies indicate how inactivity may induce tendinopathy [87, 88]; for this reason we may find, in literature, mechanical induction models of tendinopathy based on disuse. Nagawa and colleagues [89], by applying the disuse model, through suspension, on mice, observed a decrease in this surface of collagen fibers. However, the results of the experiment were nullified by the fact that the period of suspension induced a slackening of growing processes in animals which could have induced a successive slackening in the growth of collagen fibers. Since, in man, not all tendinopathies are caused by an overuse mechanism, the full comprehension of the effects of disuse of the onset of the tendinopathic phenomena could reveal great importance; for this reason, further and deeper studies are necessary in this environment.

1.5 The Iceberg Theory

In order to perfect our actual incomplete understanding of the intercurrent relationship between inflammatory phenomena and those which are more degenerative, the "Iceberg Theory" (IT) proposed by Abate and colleagues [2] seems to us of

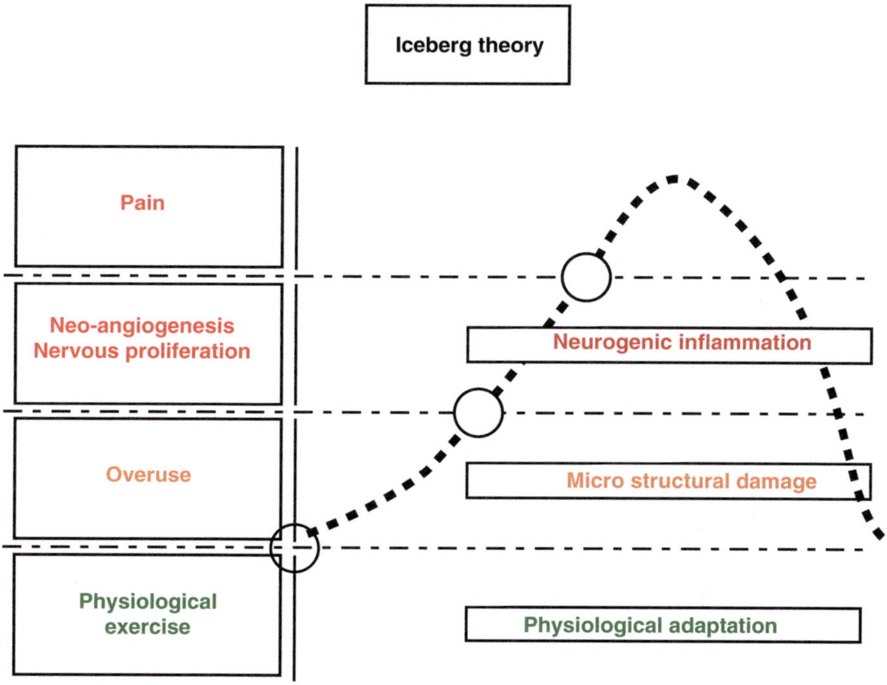

Fig. 1.1 The iceberg theory proposed by [2] allegorically illustrates the pathogenic cascade that marks the onset of tendinopathy through the levels of a hypothetical iceberg, whose base is formed by the condition of physiological normality and the tip represents the onset of the painful symptoms (From Abate et al. [2] modified)

particular interest. According to IT (Fig. 1.1), the sequence of events that follow, and which in many cases overlap, in tendinopathy may be compared to an iceberg where it is possible to see numerous levels. The base of the iceberg represents all which happens on a tendon in physiological conditions. In the initial stage of tendinopathy, we may recognize two phases: the asymptomatic phase and the symptomatic phase. This division implies that pain is the alarm symptom which marks the pathway from the first to the second phase. The first consideration is represented by the fact that it is extremely improbable that during the first phase – or shall we say non-algic – the subject undergoes an imaging examination, so the extreme base of the iceberg remains unexplored. Physical exercise, if well done and up to a certain limit, contributes in a substantial way to the increase of the mechanical resistance of the tendon, but after a certain point, we may consider likewise a true "breakpoint," and we may activate a microtraumatic mechanism which, once woken up, may lead to two different possible pictures:

1. An adequate regenerative pause may be given to the microtraumatized tendon – not necessarily by drastically diminishing physical activity but also, much more simply, by using correct workloads – such as to allow regenerative processes to prevail over the traumatic ones. In such a way, the tendon tissue maintains a functional balance.

2. An adequate regenerative pause may not be given to the microtraumatized tendon, a situation which involves a clear prevalence of tissue destruction phenomena on the regenerative ones; the tendon structure is launched toward the development of an overt tendinopathy.
   In the light of the first level iceberg exploration, we are able to draw two considerations:
   (i) The definition of tendinopathy may identify itself in a breakage of balance – existing when the tendon undergoes a physiological workload – between the auto-reparative processes and the microinjury ones.
   (ii) The borderline which marks the trespassing between physiological workload, which allows the homeostasis of the condition of the tendon, and a nonphysiological workload, responsible for the breakage of this delicate balance, is extremely unstable.

Once this existing balance has been broken between regenerative and destructive processes, and thus deviated in tendinopathy, we assist in the production of pathogenic cascade in pro-inflammatory cytokines, pro-angiogenic factors, and free radicals, which cause progressive degeneration of the tendon structure, with a possibly associated development of neural proliferation, which is responsible for the outbreak of algic symptoms.

1.6 Conclusions

The final consideration we have to make – both thanks to the amount of data of the various studies in literature and a correct and objective interpretation of the IT – is that the inflammatory and degenerative processes are not necessarily excluded but, on the contrary, may find a mutual collocation in the pathogenic cascade which distinguishes tendinopathy. So, the term tendinopathy appears more appropriate, in comparison to the definitions tendonitis and tendinosis, and able to describe the complex biological and structural rearranging, which the tendon undergoes in the case of functional sufferance.

References

1. Andres BM, Murrell GA (2008) Treatment of tendinopathy: what works, what does not, and what is on the horizon. Clin Orthop Relat Res 466(7):1539–1554
2. Abate M, Silbernagel KG, Siljeholm C, Di Iorio A, De Amicis D, Salini V, Werner S, Paganelli R (2009) Pathogenesis of tendinopathies: inflammation or degeneration? Arthritis Res Ther 11(3):235
3. Alfredson H, Ljung BO, Thorsen K, Lorentzon R (2000) In vivo investigation of ECRB tendons with microdialysis technique- no signs of inflammation but high amounts of glutamate in tennis elbow. Acta Orthop Scand 71(5):475–479

4. Alfredson H, Forsgren S, Thorsen K, Lorentzon R (2001) In vivo microdialysis and immunohistochemical analyses of tendon tissue demonstrated high amounts of free glutamate and glutamate NMDAR1 receptors, but no signs of inflammation, in Jumper's knee. J Orthop Res 19(5):881–886
5. Tallon C, Maffulli N, Ewen SW (2001) Ruptured Achilles tendons are significantly more degenerated than tendinopathic tendons. Med Sci Sports Exerc 33(12):1983–1990
6. Khan KM, Maffulli N, Coleman BD, Cook JL, Taunton JE (1998) Patellar tendinopathy: some aspects of basic science and clinical management. Br J Sports Med 32(4):346–355
7. Hashimoto T, Nobuhara K, Hamada T (2003) Pathologic evidence of degeneration as a primary cause of rotator cuff tear. Clin Orthop Relat Res 415:111–120
8. Maffulli N, Wong J, Almekinders LC (2003) Types and epidemiology of tendinopathy. Clin Sports Med 22(4):675–692
9. Kader D, Saxena A, Movin T, Maffulli N (2002) Achilles tendinopathy: some aspects of basic science and clinical management. Br J Sports Med 36(4):239–249
10. Józsa L, Kannus P (1997) Human tendon. Anatomy, physiology and pathology. In: Human Kinetics (ed) Champaign.
11. Paavola M, Kannus P, Järvinen TA, Khan K, Józsa L, Järvinen M (2002) Achilles tendinopathy. J Bone Joint Surg Am 84-A(11):2062–2076
12. Maffulli N, Sharma P, Luscombe KL (2004) Achilles tendinopathy: aetiology and management. J R Soc Med 97(10):472–476
13. Backman C, Boquist L, Fridén J, Lorentzon R, Toolanen G (1990) Chronic Achilles paratenonitis with tendinosis: an experimental model in the rabbit. J Orthop Res 8(4):541–547
14. Archambault JM, Hart DA, Herzog W (2001) Response of rabbit Achilles tendon to chronic repetitive loading. Connect Tissue Res 42(1):13–23
15. Williams IF, McCullagh KG, Goodship AE, Silver IA (1984) Studies on the pathogenesis of equine tendonitis following collagenase injury. Res Vet Sci 36(3):326–338
16. Marr CM, McMillan I, Boyd JS, Wright NG, Murray M (1993) Ultrasonographic and histopathological findings in equine superficial digital flexor tendon injury. Equine Vet J 25(1):23–29
17. Xu Y, Murrell GA (2008) The basic science of tendinopathy. Clin Orthop Relat Res 466(7):1528–1538
18. Smith MM, Sakurai G, Smith SM, Young AA, Melrose J, Stewart CM, Appleyard RC, Peterson JL, Gillies RM, Dart AJ, Sonnabend DH, Little CB (2008) Modulation of aggrecan and ADAMTS expression in ovine tendinopathy induced by altered strain. Arthritis Rheum 58(4):1055–1066
19. Yang G, Im HJ, Wang JH (2005) Repetitive mechanical stretching modulates IL-1beta induced COX-2, MMP-1 expression, and PGE_2 production in human patellar tendon fibroblasts. Gene 363:166–172
20. Varga J, Diaz-Perez A, Rosenbloom J, Jimenez SA (1987) PGE2 causes a coordinate decrease in the steady state levels of fibronectin and types I and III procollagen mRNAs in normal human dermal fibroblasts. Biochem Biophys Res Commun 147(3):1282–1288
21. Riquet FB, Lai WF, Birkhead JR, Suen LF, Karsenty G, Goldring MB (2000) Suppression of type I collagen gene expression by prostaglandins in fibroblasts is mediated at the transcriptional level. Mol Med 6(8):705–719
22. Thampatty BP, Im HJ, Wang JH (2006) Leukotriene B4 at low dosage negates the catabolic effect of prostaglandin E2 in human patellar tendon fibroblasts. Gene 372:103–109
23. Cilli F, Khan M, Fu F, Wang JH (2004) Prostaglandin E2 affects proliferation and collagen synthesis by human patellar tendon fibroblasts. Clin J Sport Med 14(4):232–236
24. Alfredson H, Pietilä T, Jonsson P, Lorentzon R (1998) Heavy-load eccentric calf muscle training for the treatment of chronic Achilles tendinosis. Am J Sports Med 26(3):360–366
25. Alfredson H, Bjur D, Thorsen K, Lorentzon R, Sandström P (2002) High intratendinous lactate levels in painful chronic Achilles tendinosis. An investigation using microdialysis technique. J Orthop Res 20(5):934–938

26. Petersen W, Pufe T, Zantop T, Tillmann B, Mentlein R (2003) Hypoxia and PDGF have a synergistic effect that increases the expression of the angiogenetic peptide vascular endothelial growth factor in Achilles tendon fibroblasts. Arch Orthop Trauma Surg 123(9):485–488
27. Pufe T, Petersen WJ, Mentlein R, Tillmann BN (2005) The role of vasculature and angiogenesis for the pathogenesis of degenerative tendons disease. Scand J Med Sci Sports 15(4):211–222
28. Sato Y, Abe M, Tanaka K, Iwasaka C, Oda N, Kanno S, Oikawa M, Nakano T, Igarashi T (2000) Signal transduction and transcriptional regulation of angiogenesis. Adv Exp Med Biol 476:109–115
29. Qi JH, Ebrahem Q, Moore N, Murphy G, Claesson-Welsh L, Bond M, Baker A, Anand-Apte B (2003) A novel function for tissue inhibitor of metalloproteinases-3 (TIMP3): inhibition of angiogenesis by blockage of VEGF binding to VEGF receptor-2. Nat Med 9(4):407–415. Epub 2003 Mar 24
30. Li Z, Yang G, Khan M, Stone D, Woo SL, Wang JH (2004) Inflammatory response of human tendon fibroblasts to cyclic mechanical stretching. Am J Sports Med 32(2):435–440
31. Almekinders LC, Banes AJ, Ballenger CA (1993) Effects of repetitive motion on human fibroblasts. Med Sci Sports Exerc 25(5):603–607
32. Wang JH, Jia F, Yang G, Yang S, Campbell BH, Stone D, Woo SL (2003) Cyclic mechanical stretching of human tendon fibroblasts increases the production of prostaglandin E2 and levels of cyclooxygenase expression: a novel in vitro model study. Connect Tissue Res 44(3-4):128–133
33. Wang JH, Li Z, Yang G, Khan M (2004) Repetitively stretched tendon fibroblasts produce inflammatory mediators. Clin Orthop Relat Res 422:243–250
34. Binderman I, Shimshoni Z, Somjen D (1984) Biochemical pathways involved in the translation of physical stimulus into biological message. Calcif Tissue Int 36(Suppl 1):S82–S85
35. Sumpio BE, Banes AJ, Link GW, Iba T (1990) Modulation of endothelial cell phenotype by cyclic stretch: inhibition of collagen production. J Surg Res 48(5):415–420
36. Brighton CT, Strafford B, Gross SB, Leatherwood DF, Williams JL, Pollack SR (1991) The proliferative and synthetic response of isolated calvarial bone cells of rats to cyclic biaxial mechanical strain. J Bone Joint Surg Am 73(3):320–331
37. Banes AJ, Tsuzaki M, Yamamoto J, Fischer T, Brigman B, Brown T, Miller L (1995) Mechanoreception at the cellular level: the detection, interpretation, and diversity of responses to mechanical signals. Biochem Cell Biol 73(7-8):349–365
38. Birukov KG, Shirinsky VP, Stepanova OV, Tkachuk VA, Hahn AW, Resink TJ, Smirnov VN (1995) Stretch affects phenotype and proliferation of vascular smooth muscle cells. Mol Cell Biochem 144(2):131–139
39. Matyas JR, Anton MG, Shrive NG, Frank CB (1995) Stress governs tissue phenotype at the femoral insertion of the rabbit MCL. J Biomech 28(2):147–157
40. Cheng GC, Libby P, Grodzinsky AJ, Lee RT (1996) Induction of DNA synthesis by a single transient mechanical stimulus of human vascular smooth muscle cells. Role of fibroblast growth factor-2. Circulation 93(1):99–105
41. Brown TD (2000) Techniques for mechanical stimulation of cells in vitro: a review. J Biomech 33(1):3–14
42. Hsieh AH, Tsai CM, Ma QJ, Lin T, Banes AJ, Villarreal FJ, Akeson WH, Sung KL (2000) Time-dependent increases in type-III collagen gene expression in medical collateral ligament fibroblasts under cyclic strains. J Orthop Res 18(2):220–227
43. Dike LE, Chen CS, Mrksich M, Tien J, Whitesides GM, Ingber DE (1999) Geometric control of switching between growth, apoptosis, and differentiation during angiogenesis using micropatterned substrates. In Vitro Cell Dev Biol Anim 35(8):441–448
44. Dirks RC, Warden SJ (2011) Models for the study of tendinopathy. J Musculoskeletal Neuronal Interact 11(2):141–149
45. Devkota AC, Weinhold PS (2005) A tissue explant system for assessing tendon overuse injury. Med Eng Phys 27(9):803–808

46. Devkota AC, Tsuzaki M, Almekinders LC, Banes AJ, Weinhold PS (2007) Distributing a fixed amount of cyclic loading to tendon explants over longer periods induces greater cellular and mechanical responses. J Orthop Res 25(8):1078–1086
47. Lavagnino M, Arnoczky SP, Tian T, Vaupel Z (2003) Effect of amplitude and frequency of cyclic tensile strain on the inhibition of MMP-1 mRNA expression in tendon cells: an in vitro study. Connect Tissue Res 44(3-4):181–187
48. Provenzano PP, Heisey D, Hayashi K, Lakes R, Vanderby R Jr (2002) Subfailure damage in ligament: a structural and cellular evaluation. J Appl Physiol 92(1):362–371
49. Wren TA, Lindsey DP, Beaupré GS, Carter DR (2003) Effects of creep and cyclic loading on the mechanical properties and failure of human Achilles tendons. Ann Biomed Eng 31(6):710–717
50. Majima T, Marchuk LL, Sciore P, Shrive NG, Frank CB, Hart DA (2000) Compressive compared with tensile loading of medial collateral ligament scar in vitro uniquely influences mRNA levels for aggrecan, collagen type II, and collagenase. J Orthop Res 18(4):524–531
51. Arnoczky SP, Tian T, Lavagnino M, Gardner K (2004) Ex vivo static tensile loading inhibits MMP-1 expression in rat tail tendon cells through a cytoskeletally based mechanotransduction mechanism. J Orthop Res 22(2):328–333
52. Warden SJ (2007) Animal model for the study of tendinopathy. Br J Sports Med 41(4):232–240
53. Foland JW, Trotter GW, Powers BE, Wrigley RH, Smith FW (1992) Effect of sodium hyaluronate in collagenase-induced superficial digital flexor tendinitis in horses. Am J Vet Res 53(12):2371–2376
54. Soslowsky LJ, Carpenter JE, DeBano CM, Banerji I, Moalli MR (1996) Development and use of an animal model for investigations on rotator cuff disease. J Shoulder Elbow Surg 5(5):383–392
55. Lui PP, Fu SC, Chan LS, Hung LK, Chan KM (2009) Chondrocyte phenotype and ectopic ossification in collagenase-induced tendon degeneration. J Histochem Cytochem 57(2):91–100
56. Fu SC, Chan KM, Chan LS, Fong DT, Lui PY (2009) The use of motion analysis to measure pain-related behaviour in a rat model of degenerative tendon injuries. J Neurosci Methods 179(2):309–318
57. Almekinders LC, Temple JD (1998) Etiology, diagnosis, and treatment of tendonitis: an analysis of the literature. Med Sci Sports Exerc 30(8):1183–1190
58. Stone D, Green C, Rao U, Aizawa H, Yamaji T, Niyibizi C, Carlin G, Woo SL (1999) Cytokine-induced tendinitis: a preliminary study in rabbits. J Orthop Res 17(2):168–177
59. Langberg H, Skovgaard D, Karamouzis M, Bülow J, Kjaer M (1999) Metabolism and inflammatory mediators in the peritendinous space measured by microdialysis during intermittent isometric exercise in humans. J Physiol 515(Pt 3):919–927
60. Sullo A, Maffulli N, Capasso G, Testa V (2001) The effects of prolonged peritendinous administration of PGE1 to the rat Achilles tendon: a possible animal model of chronic Achilles tendinopathy. J Orthop Sci 6(4):349–357
61. Khan MH, Li Z, Wang JH (2005) Repeated exposure of tendon to prostaglandin-E2 leads to localized tendon degeneration. Clin J Sport Med 15(1):27–33
62. McEwan SR, Davey PG (1988) Ciprofloxacin and tenosynovitis. Lancet 2(8616):900
63. Rose TF, Bremner DA, Collins J, Ellis-Pegler R, Isaacs R, Richardson R, Small M (1990) Plasma and dialysate levels of pefloxacin and its metabolites in CAPD patients with peritonitis. J Antimicrob Chemother 25(4):657–664
64. Lee WT, Collins JF (1992) Ciprofloxacin associated bilateral Achilles tendon rupture. Aust N Z J Med 22(5):500
65. Ribard P, Audisio F, Kahn MF, De Bandt M, Jorgensen C, Hayem G, Meyer O, Palazzo E (1992) Seven Achilles tendinitis including 3 complicated by rupture during fluoroquinolone therapy. J Rheumatol 19(9):1479–1481

66. Kato M, Takada S, Kashida Y, Nomura M (1995) Histological examination on Achilles tendon lesions induced by quinolone antibacterial agents in juvenile rats. Toxicol Pathol 23(3):385–392
67. Simonin MA, Gegout-Pottie P, Minn A, Gillet P, Netter P, Terlain B (2000) Pefloxacin-induced achilles tendon toxicity in rodents: biochemical changes in proteoglycan synthesis and oxidative damage to collagen. Antimicrob Agents Chemother 44(4):867–872
68. Kashida Y, Kato M (1997) Characterization of fluoroquinolone-induced Achilles tendon toxicity in rats: comparison of toxicities of 10 fluoroquinolones and effects of anti-inflammatory compounds. Antimicrob Agents Chemother 41(11):2389–2393
69. Williams JG (1986) Achilles tendon lesions in sport. Sports Med 3(2):114–135
70. Khan KM, Maffulli N (1998) Tendinopathy: An Achilles heel for athletes and clinicians. Clin J Sport Med 8(3):151–154
71. Möller M, Movin T, Granhed H, Lind K, Faxén E, Karlsson J (2001) Acute rupture of tendon Achilles. A prospective randomised study of comparison between surgical and non-surgical treatment. J Bone Joint Surg Br 83:843–848
72. Paavola M, Kannus P, Järvinen M (2005) Epidemiology of tendon problems in sport. In: Mafulli N, Renström P, Leadbedder W (eds) Tendon injury. Springer-Verlag London Limited, London
73. Nakama LH, King KB, Abrahamsson S, Rempel DM (2005) Evidence of tendon microtears due to cyclical loading in an in vivo tendinopathy model. J Orthop Res 23(5):1199–1205
74. Asundi KR, King KB, Rempel DM (2008) Evaluation of gene expression through qRT-PCR in cyclically loaded tendons: an in vivo model. Eur J Appl Physiol 102(3):265–270
75. Andersson G, Forsgren S, Scott A, Gaida JE, Stjernfeldt JE, Lorentzon R, Alfredson H, Backman C, Danielson P (2011) Tenocyte hypercellularity and vascular proliferation in a rabbit model of tendinopathy: contralateral effects suggest the involvement of central neuronal mechanisms. Br J Sports Med 45(5):399–406
76. Soslowsky LJ, Thomopoulos S, Tun S, Flanagan CL, Keefer CC, Mastaw J, Carpenter JE (2000) Neer Award 1999. Overuse activity injures the supraspinatus tendon in an animal model: a histologic and biomechanical study. J Shoulder Elbow Surg 9(2):79–84
77. Perry SM, McIlhenny SE, Hoffman MC, Soslowsky LJ (2005) Inflammatory and angiogenic mRNA levels are altered in a supraspinatus tendon overuse animal model. J Shoulder Elbow Surg 14(1 Suppl S):79S–83S
78. Millar NL, Wei AQ, Molloy TJ, Bonar F, Murrell GA (2009) Cytokines and apoptosis in supraspinatus tendinopathy. J Bone Joint Surg Br 91(3):417–424
79. Huang TF, Perry SM, Soslowsky LJ (2004) The effect of overuse activity on Achilles tendon in an animal model: a biomechanical study. Ann Biomed Eng 32(3):336–341
80. Glazebrook MA, Wright JR Jr, Langman M, Stanish WD, Lee JM (2008) Histological analysis of Achilles tendons in an overuse rat model. J Orthop Res 26(6):840–846
81. Lindstedt SL, LaStayo PC, Reich TE (2001) When active muscles lengthen: properties and consequences of eccentric contractions. News Physiol Sci 16:256–261
82. Ljungqvist R (1967) Subcutaneous partial rupture of the Achilles tendon. Acta Orthop Scand Suppl 113:1–5
83. Fridén J (1984) Muscle soreness after exercise: implications of morphological changes. Int J Sports Med 5(2):57–66
84. Stauber WT, Clarkson PM, Fritz VK, Evans WJ (1990) Extracellular matrix disruption and pain after eccentric muscle action. J Appl Physiol 69(3):868–874
85. Sun HB, Li Y, Fung DT, Majeska RJ, Schaffler MB, Flatow EL (2008) Coordinate regulation of IL-1beta and MMP-13 in rat tendons following subrupture fatigue damage. Clin Orthop Relat Res 466(7):1555–1561
86. Fung DT, Wang VM, Andarawis-Puri N, Basta-Pljakic J, Li Y, Laudier DM, Sun HB, Jepsen KJ, Schaffler MB, Flatow EL (2010) Early response to tendon fatigue damage accumulation in a novel in vivo model. J Biomech 43(2):274–279

87. Rolf C, Movin T (1997) Etiology, histopathology, and outcome of surgery in achillodynia. Foot Ankle Int 18(9):565–569
88. Alfredson H, Lorentzon R (2000) Chronic Achilles tendinosis: recommendations for treatment and prevention. Sports Med 29(2):135–146
89. Nakagawa Y, Totsuka M, Sato T, Fukuda Y, Hirota K (1989) Effect of disuse on the ultrastructure of the Achilles tendon in rats. Eur J Appl Physiol Occup Physiol 59(3):239–242

Chapter 2
Healing Processes of the Tendon

Gian Nicola Bisciotti and Piero Volpi

Abstract The biological principles on which the healing process of the tendon is based are quite different from the biological principles that regulate the muscle healing process, although some aspects may be considered as similar. Especially the last stage, namely, the remodeling and maturation phases, is very different especially regarding the temporal length that in the tendon, in respect to the muscle, is much greater. However the healing process between the tendon and the muscle will not only differ in the length time. In effect, the extrinsic and intrinsic healing mechanisms are a peculiar feature of the tendon healing that have no similarity with what occurs in the muscle during its healing process. Therefore it is of fundamental importance, especially after tendon surgical treatment, to know the biological principles that guide the healing process of the tendon.

2.1 Introduction

For a better understanding of the biological principles on which the healing process of the tendon is based, we are going to make a brief yet detailed review, in this chapter, on the various healing phases of the tendon tissue after undergoing injury or surgery. The full comprehension in a biological sense of these different phases makes up the absolutely necessary introduction to be able to fully understand etiology and the development of tissue disorder on the tendon tissue and the pathways

G.N. Bisciotti
Qatar Orthopaedic and Sports Medicine Hospital, FIFA Center of Excellence, Doha, Qatar
e-mail: bisciotti@libero.it

P. Volpi (✉)
Humanitas Clinical Institute, IRCCS, Rozzano, Milan, Italy

FC Internazionale Medical staff, Milan, Italy
e-mail: volpi.piero@libero.it

G.N. Bisciotti, P. Volpi (eds.), *The Lower Limb Tendinopathies*,
Sports and Traumatology, DOI 10.1007/978-3-319-33234-5_2

which may compromise the complete anatomical and functional recovery. Such theoretical base is, and thus the prerequisite, to be able to put into practice efficient strategies whose aim is the streamlining of the natural healing processes of healing the tendon. The healing process of the tendon tissue, on the other hand, as all other soft tissues, may essentially base itself on three biological principles or the regeneration, the repair, or a combination of both. Regeneration represents a form of biological healing which comes about through the production of new tissue whose structural and fundamental characteristics are identical to those of the primitive tissue [1]. Tissue regeneration would therefore represent, in theory, the ideal healing process for the injured soft tissues, exactly as in the case of the skeletal muscle [3]; the healing of the tendon tissue comes about thanks to a repair process which shows itself in the formation of a more or less conspicuous scarring area, which once again, exactly as in the case of the skeletal muscle, presents itself of connective nature and with structural and functional properties inferior to those of original tissue [4]. The tendon tissue, in comparison with the muscular one, presents reduced self-repairing capacity given by the scarce vascularity which, in its turn, involves a reduced amount of oxygen and nutriment of tissue, even though some authors sustain that the self-repairing processes of the tendon are, however, underestimated [5–7].

From a general point of view, the process of tendon repair is divided into the same phases in which the repair process of the skeletal muscle is structured, or into three consecutive phases but, at the same time, extremely interconnected, which are:

- The inflammatory phase, which begins in immediate injury, which is prolonged until about the fourth to the seventh day
- The proliferative phase, which starts from the end of the first post-injury week until the fourth–sixth week
- The maturing or remodeling phase, which from the end of the proliferative phase may prolong itself for up to 1 year from the outbreak of injury

As in the case of muscle tissue repair, the pathway from one phase to another is extremely soft, creating pictures of biological coexistence between the two considered phases. Let us consider now the different biological stages before briefly describing them in their principle details.

2.2 The Inflammatory Phase

The inflammatory phase, also called the exudative phase, begins in the immediate post-trauma period as a physiological answer of structural damage. Following the damage in the vascular network, blood, plasma, and tissue fluids are spilt inside the injured area. The platelets present in the injured area link with collagen exposed by trauma and release phospholipids which stimulate the mechanisms of coagulation [8]. About an hour after trauma in the injured area, we may observe fibrin and fibronectin which form cross-links with the injured collagen fibers [9, 10]. Already, these first stages bring about the formation of a tenuous glue-like structure which acts as a real "cork," even though still structurally fragile, which in any case banks the local hemorrhage and mechanically supports the damaged tendon fibers when supporting the tensile strengths, which they undergo during this first post-injury phase. In a few hours, a large migration of leukocytes of the injured area comes about, polymorphonucleates and monocytes. Such cellular infiltration happens before 24 h from the trauma and carries on for the next 2–3 days. The inflammatory phase represents a relatively short time, about 1 week [8, 11, 12] The cellular elements, the polymorphonucleates leukocytes, the monocytes, and the macrophages migrate inside the injured area, attracted by particular substances produced inside the injured area, named chemotactic agents. Among these substances, histamine stands out, a substance which is released by mastocytes, granular leukocytes, and platelets. Histamine performs a vasodilator action, increasing the vascular permeability. Still among the chemotactic substances, fibronectin also stands out, which performs a chemotactic action on the leukocytes and the macrophages, and bradykinin, which, as well as increasing vascular permeability, stimulates the releasing of prostaglandin during the inflammatory stage. This latter one is influenced by prostaglandins, in particular prostaglandin E (PGE) which increases vascular permeability and the prostaglandin E2 (PGE2) which has the capacity to attract leukocytes. Immediately after injury we may also observe a rapid increase of DNA inside tendon cells, which then stabilizes itself in the following phases of proliferation, of remodeling, and of maturation [13–15]. In the later period of the inflammatory phase, the PGE and the PGE2 may start up a precocious process of repairing, continuing, and, at the same time, the inflammatory reaction, providing a first example of how the various phases are often overlapping. One of the main tasks of the pro-inflammatory cells is to remove necrotic and refuse produce from the injured area; only after these have been removed, or after 5–7 days from the injury, the proliferative phase may fully begin. As we have already mentioned, a clear subdivision between the inflammatory phase, the proliferative phase, and the last phase of maturation does not exist; however, we may observe rather a continuum of biological activity, which presents overlapping aspects [8]. Several studies have suggested how the different characteristics, which the inflammatory phase may assume, are crucial for success, or, on the contrary, for the failing of the healing processes of the tendon [16]. For example, on an animal model, neutropenia accelerates the healing process from cut injuries [16] but does not influence the healing processes of a tendon which has been surgically repaired [17]. The depletion of the macrophages compromises the healing processes of the skin, causing both diminution of the processes of collagen deposition and angiogenesis [18, 19]. However, this discussion in literature data is contrasting; in fact, on the one hand, several authors indicate that the activation of macrophages may represent new and interesting therapeutic approaches on tissue repair, for example, regarding damage on cardiac tissue in the case of ischemia [20]; on the other hand, other studies indicate that the depletion of the macrophages implies a substantial improvement both of the morphology and of the mechanical properties of the interfacial tendon bone after surgical reconstruction of LCA [21]. This incomplete comprehension of the role of neutrophils and macrophages in the process of tissue reparation may be, at least in part, justified by the fact that during the inflammatory phase, a molecule may adhere to various function and, at the same time, different molecules may perform substantially overlapping roles [22]. Taking this into consideration, it is opportune to remember that the different grades of the severity of the injury may determine different states of activation of the macrophages [23, 24] or:

(i) A first type of activation named "innate," triggered by lipopolysaccharides or by interferon-γ (IFN-γ)-inducing factor (IGIF) associated with the pro-inflammatory state and the production of interleukin 6 (IL-6), interleukin 1-β (IL-1β), and tumor necrosis factor-α (TNF-α)
(ii) A second mode of inflammation called "classic" activated by the action of IL-4 and IL-23 associated with the action of TGF-β, TGF-α, basic fibroblastic growth factor (b-FGF), PDGF, and VEGF.

In fact, several studies, even though preliminary, indicate a high level of complexity in the activation of macrophages, a level which depends on the nature of interaction and from the combination of biological stimulus to which the same macrophages are exposed [25]. The resolution of the inflammatory processes is, in the end, regulated by the fibroblast activity, which contributes in a substantial way, allowing the infiltrated leukocytes both to move toward apoptosis processes and to leave the tissue through the lymphatic circle [26]. Furthermore, several studies which report the observation of an increase in mastocytes during the inflammatory phase in patients affected by chronic tendinopathy with evident vascular hyperplasia and who complained about excel algic symptoms must be noticed [27, 28]. Since mastocytes contain numerous granules rich in heparin, histamine, and tryptase,[1] the release of these last two substances on behalf of the mastocytes during the degranulation phase participate in the release of substance B, which is responsible for the algic symptoms [27–29].

2.3 The Proliferative Phase

The proliferative phase begins with an accumulation of fibroblasts, myofibroblasts,[2] and endothelial cells inside the injury area [30–33]. The processes of migration and proliferation of these cells are promoted by the presence of growth factors produced both by the platelets and by macrophages [8]. Proliferation of new capillaries commences in this stage, which begin to functionally communicate with the

[1] *Tryptase is a proteolytic enzyme present in mast cell granules.*

[2] *The myofibroblasts are connective tissue cells with contractile capabilities similar to the smooth muscle. Discovered in 1970, at these cells, an important role is recognized in the process of wound healing, tissue fibrosis, and pathological fascia contractures. Their evolution generally occurs from normal fibroblasts to proto-myofibroblasts, until the complete differentiation into myofibroblasts and to end to a terminal apoptosis that is influenced by mechanical tension, cytokines, and specific proteins from the extracellular matrix.*

pre-existing capillary network. During the proliferative phase, the fibroblasts and the myofibroblasts, which may come from the same tendon, from the epitenon, from the tendon sheath, and from paratenon [34], show a strong proliferative activity and a synthesis of the extracellular matrix components (ECM). An important role is played by the b-FGF above all regarding the cellular proliferation and the vascularity inside the injured area [35]. The interaction between neoformed capillary fibroblasts and myofibroblasts and ECM give origin to the granulation tissue, and the original "cork" of glue-like substance, formed in the first stages of the inflammatory phase, is substituted by a more stable structure. At the same time, fibronectin makes the migration and the adhesion of fibroblasts better. In the initial stage of the proliferative phase, more precisely starting from the seventh day of the injury, The fibroblasts produce glycosaminoglycans of the ECM (mainly hyaluronic acid) and collagen type III, even if a clear increase of the synthesis of collagen is observable only from the post-injury third week. The new collagen fibers which form possess, however, neither a consistent organizational structure nor a clear anatomical orientation. The last period of the proliferative phase registers the production of collagen type I, which continues until the end of the maturation and remodeling phases [2]. Collagen type I starting at about the 12th to 14th day begins to substitute collagen type III, and in the meantime, the granulation tissue is further maturing, and the scar formation assumes its solidity structure. During this phase, we may observe a decrease in the activity of the oxidative enzymes and a clear increase of the anaerobic enzymes [4]. It is interesting to note that also in the injured skeletal muscle in a few hours from injury, the consumption of oxygen at rest, inside the injured muscle, heightens dramatically, generating an imbalance between the refueling and the request of O_2, which determines a rapid descent of the tension of O_2 inside the insulted area; contextually we assist in an increase of the lactate concentrate inside the injury. The proliferative phase in the tendon lasts approximately from 3 to 6 weeks, a period which is progressively substituted by the maturation and remodeling phases.

2.4 The Remodeling and Maturation Phases

This latter one is temporally the longer one; it may go on for 1 year from the injury [8]. During the remodeling phase, the number of macrophages, fibroblasts, myoblasts, and capillaries diminishes in a slow and progressive way and contextually also the activity of synthesis drops. The scar area becomes less dense, its capillarity decreases, and also its matrix loses a certain fluidity; in the phase we assist, at first, in a progressive substitution of the reparation granular tissue on behalf of the fibrous tissue and, from the tenth week onward, a further substitution of the fibrous tissue on behalf of the tendon tissue [36]. Also the quantity of the glycosaminoglycans slowly decreases, changing its own distribution. The tendon collagen becomes less dense in its structural compactness and is mainly composed of collagen type I. In all, during this last third phase, we assist in a remodeling of the neoformed collagen fibers, until the latter ones do not form a strong permanent structure [1, 2]. The full maturation of the collagen and a total realignment of the fibers usually need a period of 5 or 6 months from the outbreak of the injury. Toward the end of the remodeling phase, the fibroblasts, ceasing their biosynthetic activity, transform themselves into fibrocytes. In spite of this large remodeling process, the biomechanical and biochemical losses following the trauma may indefinitely maintain themselves [1, 2, 37]. The tensile strength of the tendon may reduce itself to over 30 % [1, 2, 37], and the structure of the latter may present defects in the distribution of collagen with an increase of collagen type III and V at the expense of that of type I, of the positioning of the fibers, and of the content in water, DNA, and proteoglycans [33]. It is interesting to note that the mechanism just described is represented by the proteolysis process. The proteolithic activity, in fact, results as a biological component essential for both tissue growth and its maintenance, not to mention of its adaptation and reparation processes. After an injury the proteolysis becomes necessary both for the removal of the damaged matrix and for the remodeling of the scar area [38].

2.5 The Role of the Nervous Response in the Healing Processes of the Tendon

Following trauma, of any nature, the initial stress of the organism is codified in a neural sign [26]. Despite the fact that the tendon is essentially lacking in its own nervous component [39], the unmyelinated axons which innervate the peritenon and the endotenon receive molecular products coming from the injury and, thus, transmit a recorded signal in order to modulate the efferent neural response with the immune response [40] So, the nervous system plays a fundamental role in the regulation of the processes of tendon reparation; this shows the fact that the application of calcitonin gene-related peptide (CGRP), of substance P [40–42], or of nerve growth factor (NGF) [43] improves in an animal model, the process of repairing the tendon, whereas denervation, both in mice and rabbits [44], respectively, worsens and delays the processes of tissue repair of the medial collateral ligament and Achilles tendon. In fact, obviously, a denerved anatomical system does not possess a physiological potential such as to allow it to face the integration request of the various and multiple biological requests coming from tissue in a reparation phase. On the other hand, also the scarce repairing capability of cartilage is substantially due to its un-neural and un-vascular nature [45]. The nerves and the blood vessels therefore adopt a synergic strategy of reciprocated support in the repairing of the tendon. In mice, for example, we may observe how nerves and vessels proliferate together from the peritenon during the proliferative phase, whereas during the remodeling phase, we may observe a strong neo-innervation in the surrounding areas in comparison with the area of repair tissue. This neo-innervation aims at reducing angiogenesis during the same remodeling phase [39].

2.6 The Role of the Apoptosis Process in the Last Stage of the Healing of the Tendon

The return of a normal situation of homeostasis tissue after injury is conditioned by a clearance of neoformed fibroblasts [47]. The density of the fibroblasts normally grows up until the fourth post-injury day to then decrease in a constant way. In each case, during the healing processes of the tendon, the density of the fibroblasts remains high by a percentage equal to 6–7 times the base value. This notable increase of the fibroblast activity is justified by the fact that the fibroblasts cover a fundamental role in the depositing and remodeling processes of ECM; however, this also indicates the biological necessity that such events return to normality at the end of the healing process of the tendon. Some authors hypothesize that this downregulation comes about, thanks to apoptosis phenomenon, a process characterized by the condensation of chromatin, fragmentation, formation of mass around the cellular casing, and destruction of the cytoskeleton [47–49]. All these phenomena show in a contraction of nuclear casing and of the cellular membrane, driving the cell to programmed self-elimination. The apoptotic cells are then removed by a silent physiological mechanism where the role of the central regulator is carried out by caspasis (a group of protease which contain cysteine in the active site). A certain number of studies witness the existence of the apoptotic phenomenon in tendon fibroblasts both on man and animals, in vivo and in vitro [49–51]. Both electromagnetic fields [52] and the oxidative stress [53] and the fluoroquinolones [54] are able to provoke the apoptosis phenomenon on tendon fibroblasts in culture. In the animal model, the rate of apoptosis appears very low in a structurally and biologically healthy tendon (range 0.56–1.3 %) [51], whereas it appears much higher in the case of tendinopathy [55]. On the contrary, in samples of human tendons devoid of disease, we may observe a particularly high amount of apoptotic cells, with an index of about 35 % in active remodeling sites and on average 26 % of tenocytes [56]. Since the ratio of apoptosis in tendon tissue, affected by tendinopathy, does not differ to that observed in a healthy tendon, or, to say 34 % versus 35 % [56], we may reasonably suppose that, in man, the apoptotic phenomenon is naturally linked to the normal turnover of tendon cells inside which we find the most complex remodeling process of ECM and that such a process may be seen in both normal and pathological conditions. In a pathologic picture represented by the healing process of the tendon, apoptosis is involved in the clearance mechanism of the excessive proliferation of fibroblasts which may be seen in the site of injury repair. The apoptosis phenomenon during the process of tendon repair, as witnessed in the caspasis activity, shows starting from the 14th day to then, it reaches its peak around the 28th post-injury day, even if some authors form the hypothesis that the apoptosis may be mediated also by other proteins in comparison with those of caspasis [46, 57]. The apoptosis interests not only the fibroblasts but also the myofibroblasts which disappear, because of the latter, in the final phase of healing [58, 59]. Apoptosis is a fairly rapid process, which requires from just a few minutes up to 1 h, and so reveals difficulty in sample testing, seeing as some cells may respond quicker than others. It is probably for this reason we may explain the relative lack of studies and the consequent necessity for further analysis in this area. However, given that the cellular density of the tendon at the end of its repairing processes, it may be established by the ratio between the growth and the death of cells which may be seen in the injured area, the ability to deepen the knowledge of the processes which regulates such a phenomenon, and first of all apoptosis, it allows us to fully comprehend the mechanisms which permit the tendon tissue to reach a new situation of homeostasis once the repairing processes have been completed.

2.7 The Role of Growth Factors in the Healing Process of the Tendon

The growth factors (GF) assume a very important role inside the various phases of the healing process of the tendon, a role based on their specific operating target and their heterochronism action. The full understanding of how and when the various GF and their receptors in the process of tendon repair may be expressed by representing a future and most important stage in research by optimizing the processes of tendon tissue repair. We may thus resume the role and the timing of the GF in the course of the three stages of tendon tissue repair:

The platelet-derived growth factor (PDGF) is only produced for a short time immediately after the injury and stimulates the other GF [60, 61].

The transforming growth factor-beta (TGF-ß) is active during the inflammatory and proliferative phases but assumes an even more important role during the second of the said phases. By separately analyzing its three isoforms, we may observe how the TGF-ß contributes to the sedimentation of ECM and how its overexpression appears in the formation of fibrotic tissue; furthermore it is possible to note how TGF- ß2 acts in a similar way to that of TGF-ß1 and that in the end TGF-ß3 shows the capacity to improve the scar tissue. The peak of the activity of the receptors of the expression of TGF-ß is registered around the 14th post-injury day and begins to decrease by around the 56th day [62–64].

The vascular endothelial growth factor (VEGF) stimulates the proliferation of endothelial cells, improves the angiogenesis, and increases the capillary permeability. Inside the injured area, the expression of VEGF RNA may be observed from the seventh post-injury day, whereas its peak is registered around the tenth day [65, 66].

The isoforms of nitric oxide synthase (NOS)[3] are expressed, through different expression patterns, during all three phases of tendon repair [67] (Table 2.1).

[3] *NO synthase is an enzyme distributed almost ubiquitously in tissues and in living organism in general that provides to produce NO starting from arginine that is converted to citrulline (intermediate metabolite of the urea cycle).*

Table 2.1 Diagram of the main cellular alterations and of the matrix regarding the reparation period

Period	Main cellular and matrix alterations
Immediately after injury	The presence of erythrocytes often grouped together in the form of small clots. Presence of fibronectin (within 1 h) and macrophages
24 h later	The presence of polymorphonuclear leukocytes, monocytes, and macrophages (also before in case of mechanical breakage and later on case of spontaneous breakage) Beginning of the synthesis of hyaluronic acid, followed by the synthesis of glycosaminoglycans (in any case later on)
Fourth to fifth day	The presence of fibroblasts
From the seventh day onward	Slow and progressive diminution of leukocytes, macrophages, and fibroblast activity Increase in the presence of fibronectin No presence of procollagen before the seventh day From the seventh day, collagen synthesis begins in the epitenon but not still in the endotenocytes The presence of myofibroblasts in the granulation tissue
Second week	The granulation tissue becomes more compact The fibroblasts (tenoblasts) show orientation on the main axis of the tendon The collagen synthesis is evident also in areas detached from the repair zone The neoformed collagen type III (formed in the injured zone) is progressively substituted by collagen type I (formed outside the injured area) A progressive increase in tensile strength of the tendon begins with the substitution from collagen type I to type III
Fourth week	The number of fibroblasts, myofibroblasts, and capillaries starts to decrease The number of macrophages clearly diminishes Collagen forms dense packages of fibers
From the fourth week onward	The remodeling and maturation phases continue, which may carry on for a period between 4 and 11 months

2.8 The Role of Angiogenesis in Cellular Proliferation

The high concentration of GF and cytokines secreted at first by the platelets and the leukocytes followed by the macrophages produces a rapid increase in several specific cellular populations, like endothelial cells, migrant fibroblasts, and resident tendon cells. Above all, it is important to note that the number of tenocytes contextually increases the phenomenon of angiogenesis [26]. In an animal model, the VEGF-A is precociously present in the post-traumatic phase of tendon damage [68], whereas others just as important GF for proliferation and vascular stability (like TGF-β, PDGF-BB, and angiopoietin-1) are observable inside the injury only in the following phases [69].

2.9 The Intrinsic and Extrinsic Healing Processes of the Tendon

Several authors sustain the hypothesis that the healing processes of the tendon have origin from the two injured tendon stumps. This theory is called "the theory of intrinsic healing." Other studies, instead, attribute tendon healing to the sole cellular activity in peritenon tissue. This second theory is known as "theory of extrinsic healing." In the end, a third thought is to recognize the two aforementioned processes as an equally complemented role.

2.9.1 Extrinsic Healing Mechanisms

Since 1962 [70] showed that in a cut tendon, repaired by suturing and thus immobilized, the reparation came about thanks to the formation of granular tissue coming from the peritendon structures, where an intense proliferative activity was observable. During this repairing process on the peritendon, the author observed that the tendon tissue remained inert and following this observation concluded that the tendon tissue was missing in any type of repair capacity whatsoever. So, the total loss of self-reparative properties of the tendon tissue should show its healing processes which entirely entrust the formation of scars. Other authors hypothesize that during the reparative process of the tendon, the phenomenon of neovascularity has origin mainly from the paratenon and other peritendon tissues and that its own vascularity has a minor role [71]. Also other authors [72] support this hypothesis, confirming that tendon repair processes come about through the surrounding tenosynovia in the area where the fibroblast cells cover the injury on the tendon body. However, an obvious observation regarding this affirmation is in the fact that one of the main causes of failure in the recuperation of full tendon functionality following a breakage is represented by the formation of scars between the suture area and the peritendinous structures [73]. So, the fact that extrinsic repair of the tendon bases itself on the formation of adherence, and, at the same time, these latter ones strongly limit the full recovery of the tendon flow represents an oxymoron [74]. Indeed, from the moment that full functionality of a tendon depends largely on its flow capacity, the peritendinous adherences, very often, have to be surgically removed. In the specific case of the Achilles tendon, we must remember that, since it presents reduced movement, the eventual formation of adherences does not limit its functionality in a dramatic way, as however happens in the case of finger tendons, which, on the other hand, present a much more ample movement [75, 76].

2.9.2 Intrinsic Healing Mechanisms

Even before the studies of Potenza [70], Wheeldon [77] referred to how the use of a cellophane membrane to rebuild the flow sheath after suturing the long extensor tendon of the thumb obtained full anatomical healing of the tendon and a total recovery of its functionality without the formation of peritendinous adherences. Further studies confirmed the capacity of intrinsic repair in the tendon tissue, both in breakages of the flexor tendons of man [73, 74] and animals in vivo and in vitro [14, 15, 78–80]. All these studies showed the intrinsic healing capacity on behalf of the tendon, both in vivo and in vitro, based on experiments which foresaw, during the repair process of the tendon, the exclusion of all possible external cellular contributions such as circulation and the influence of synovial liquid. In such a situation, phagocytosis comes about through the transformation of epitenon fibroblasts, whereas the synthesis of collagen is mainly performed by the endotenon cells, whose migration on the injured tendon has been observed also in an in vivo model [81, 82]. In all studied models, the nutritive contribution necessary for tendon healing processes is provided by the synovial fluid, and repair comes about without the formation of adherences. In normal clinical practice, on the contrary, the lysis of the tendon adherences is necessary in 20–30 % of cases [76]. The diatribe between the sustainers of the mechanisms of extrinsic and intrinsic repair may substantially settle by keeping the hypothesis that the intra-tendon micro-circle, and the production of synovial fluid is preserved thanks to the type of surgery used, and if, at the same time, the injured tendon is immobilized in time (compatible with its repair processes), the tenocytes are able to genetically express a self-repairing program and thus give life to intrinsic repair. If instead, the nutritive contribution of the tendon, following surgical repair is jeopardized the mechanisms of extrinsic repair may prevail over those of intrinsic repair above all if we add an excessive immobilization period [83, 84]. In any case , we must remember that the precise effects of mechanical stimulation of a tendon in repair in man are still not clear [85].

2.10 The Molecular Bases of Neoformation of the Tendon

Even though no markers of the tendon morphogenesis have been indicated as a potential target of the neoformation processes of the tendon, evidence exists that such a process may be influenced by the activation of specific factors. The factors which have the most documentation in this area are the growth and differentiation factors (GDFs) and scleraxis (Scx).[4] The GDFs represent a group of the superfamily of transforming growth factor-β – bone morphogenetic protein (TGF-β/BMP) and are secreted in the form of mature peptides which form homo and heterodimers[5] [86]. Initially some studies have shown how the GDFs, the GDF6 and the GDF7 were, in

---

[4] *The protein scleraxis (Locus: Chr. 8 q24.3) is a member of the superfamily of transcription factors basic helix-loop-helix (bHLH). It is expressed in mature tendons and ligaments of the limbs and trunk but also in their progenitors. The gene coding for Scx is expressed in all the connective tissues that mediate the connection of the muscle to the bone structure, as well as in their progenitors that are found in primitive mesenchyme.*

[5] *A dimer is a molecule formed by the union of two subunits (called monomers) of an identical chemical nature (homodimer) or of a chemical nature different (heterodimer).*

mice, implicated in the processes of osteogenesis through endochondral ossification or the bone formation that begins with the condensation of mesenchymal cells [67, 87]. The first studies which identified a marker of articular development in mice in the GDF5 go back to 1996 [88]. In these experiments the authors showed how GDF5 were necessary and sufficient for the cartilage development process on animals. In mice the role of GDF5 in tendon formation on subjects which had tendon abnormalities has recently shown, for example, an insufficient development of the patellar tendon, due to structural alterations of collagen [89]. Even more recently [90] it has been observed, in mice and in subjects which present a deficiency of GDF5, an incomplete development of femoral condyles and of intra-articular ligaments of the knee. Regarding this, it is interesting to observe that, in studied subjects, a large and excessive apoptosis of mesenchymal cells in the area of development of the knee articulation has been seen. However, if both these studies show, with sufficient evidence, the role taken on by GDFs in the development of articulation, otherwise may not be said regarding the morphogenesis of the tendons. We must, however, remember that a study by Wolfman and coll. [91] had already shown that the expression of human GDF5, GDF6, and GDF7 in ectopic sites in adult animals induced the formation of connective tissue rich in collagen of type I similar to the neoformation of tendon and ligament tissue. Furthermore, Wolfman and coll. [91] observed that the co-implant, intramuscular or subcutaneous of GDF5, GDF6, and GDF7 with BPM-2, induces the formation, in a tissue containing contextually bone and tendon tissue, suggesting in such a way that the GDFs perform a tenogenic effect also in the presence of BMP-2 and in osteogenic conditions. More recent studies [92] also use the hypothesis that the GDFs have, on an adult animal, a stimulating effect on the regeneration and the neoformation of the tendon, as well as in the tendon morphogenesis on animals in development. The administration of human recombining GDFs (rhGDF5) in the injured area of a sutured tendon in mice induces a significant improvement of the healing processes, which results in a higher tensile strength and in stiffness of the tendon compared with the counter-lateral, equally cut and sutured, but which has not received the administration on rhGDF5 [92]. To obtain an effective improvement of soft injured tissue through growth factors (e.g., GDF5 in the case of tendon tissue), a crucial point is represented by the full comprehension of all the temporary sequence of events which happen during the natural healing processes of the various types of tissue considered. In the specific case of the tendon, when it undergoes a structural injury, we assist in the formation of a hematoma in the injured area which works as a matrix for the following invasion on behalf of the mesenchymal cells which, as we know, carry out a determining role in the processes of tissue repair [85]. The injecting of GDFs inside the hematoma during the formation phase has been considered by some authors as a promising therapeutic approach able to improve tendon healing processes [93]. The administration of transgenic GDF5 through an adenoviral vector in the area of the Achilles tendon in mice shows an improvement in terms of caliber and strength of the repaired tendon, if compared to the counter-lateral which has not received GDF5 [94]. It is, however, important to underline the fact that the authors, during said experimentation, observed an abnormal proliferation of cartilage tissue inside the formed repaired tendon tissue, a fact which indicates possible disturbance of the repair processes of GDF5. We may, anyway, assume from the various available studies on the argument that GDF5 may be considered as a reasonable candidate regarding the tendon neoformation and the possible improvement of tissue repair processes. In spite of this, the fact that GDF5 in vivo may induce bone and cartilage neoformation could prevent the use of a factor of tendon regeneration [95, 96, 97]. However, since the effects of GDFs are, in mice, of dose-dependent type (300 μg of rhGDF5 induces bone and cartilage formation, whereas 500 μg only provokes bone formation), maybe it is possible that fine regulation of the dose may be the key to the solution of the problem, allowing an improvement of tendon tissue in healing, excluding the formation of other undesired neo-tissues. As well as GDFs, much research also indicates Scx as a possible molecule marker of the processes of tendon neoformation. The protein Scx (scleraxis-locus: Chr. 8 q24.3) is a member of the superfamily of transcription factors basic helix-loop-helix (bHLH) and is expressed in mature tendons and in ligaments of the limbs and the trunk but also in their pro-parents. The gene which codifies for Scx is expressed in all connective tissues which mediate the connection of the muscle to bone structure, as well as in their pro-parents which are found in the primitive mesenchymal. Scx is the best marker of tendon morphogenesis, and there is growing evidence on the fact that it can cover the same role also regarding the processes of tendon neoformation. As already mentioned, Scx is a bHLH transcription factor [98], and it may link to DNA sequences containing the "E-box[6]" consensus sequence[7] though it is bHLH [98]. During embryogenesis in mice, the transcription of Scx is observable both in areas of formation of pro-parent tendons and in the somite[8] of the same pro-parent tendons called sindetoma [99]. The analysis of sequence of Scx shows the presence of all the amino acids which characterize the bHLH[9] family [100]; however, other residues of the base regions are different in comparison with other transcription factors of bHLH, suggesting, in such a way, that Scx ties a specific group of E-box [100]. So, despite the fact that in pro-parent tendons, or in other bone and cartilage structures, an important formation of collagen type I and II is required, we may observe high levels of Scx transcription, whose role would seem limited to the function of progenitor tendons [99]. Scx is expressed in anatomical sites similar

---

[6] *An E-box is a DNA sequence that is typically located upstream of a gene in a "promoter region."*

[7] *In molecular biology and bioinformatics, a "consensus sequence" refers to the most common amino acid or nucleotide in a particular position after more aligned sequences.*

[8] *Somite [from the Greek "soma," body-ite], in embryology, is each of the segments in which it divides the dorsal mesoderm (or epimer), left and right of the spinal column. The somites give rise to elements that will form the dermis of the skin of the trunk (dermatomes), the muscles (myotomes), and the axial skeleton (sclerotomi).*

[9] *The myogenic regulatory factors are transcription factors belonging to the family "basic helix-loop-helix" (bHLH), because they contain a basic domain involved in binding to the DNA and a domain HLH needed to form homodimers or heterodimers with other proteins containing HLH domains. The bHLH motif is found in many transcription factors that are ubiquitously expressed in a tissue-specific manner.*

to those in which we observe the expression MyoD[10] which determines muscular morphogenesis. This would suggest that Scx acts in the area of tendon development in close association with the phenomenon of muscular development but without overlapping the action of MyoD [99]. This represents an important aspect of research in the area of factors which can improve the tendon healing processes, because it is obvious that the choice does not necessarily fall on the molecular target which does not imply, at the same time, muscular neoformation.

Even though many studies demonstrate an active role of Scx in tendon morphogenesis, it is still not evident that this may induce the phenomenon of tendon neoformation. Scx ties to the E-box consensus sequence as a heterodimer with E12 (a member of the family of E proteins which forms heterodimers with the bHLH protein and ties to DNA to regulate the genic expression). Furthermore, Scx is a powerful trans-activator of the genic expression [100]. A study by Lèjard and coll. [101] shows how Scx regulates the expression of the codifying gene for collagen type I in the fibroblasts of the tendon, or the COL1A1. In a recent experiment, done on mutant homozygous mice for an invalid allele Scx (Scx mice), we observed a strong disturbance of the processes of differentiation and of tendon formation [102]. The severity of the disturbance in these processes was variable, in some cases reaching a true destructive phenomenon, whereas in others, the tendon unity remained substantially intact. This study would thus use the observation previously executed by Lèjard and coll. [101] and would confirm the fact that Scx would activate the expression of the genes involved in tendon development even though the exact functions of such mechanisms remains, for now, unknown. So, we may conclude that the transcription factor bHLH Scx may, in all effect, be considered as an important marker of tendon neoformation; thus its involvement in neoformation processes also uses the hypothesis that Scx, once activated, would be able to induce the regeneration of tendon tissue, even though such an affirmation is today missing in sufficient evidence.

2.11 Conclusions

The processes of tendon repair, even though they largely trace the stages of skeletal muscle repair, maintain their specificity, differing themselves from a muscular model under numerous and non-under-valuating aspects. For example, the mechanisms of intrinsic and extrinsic healing represent a peculiarity of the mechanisms of tissue repair of the tendon, which do not find analogy in the healing processes of the skeletal muscle. For this reason, the rehabilitation process of the injured tendon is completely different from that applicable in the case of muscle injury. Also, the process of tendon neoformation in the adult covers fundamental importance, above all considering the fact that their optimization could resolve the long-standing

[10] *The MyoD gene encoding a transcription factor involved in the differentiation of the muscle, in particular, induces fibroblasts to differentiate into myoblasts.*

problem of the healing of tendon tissue, a problem which today has still not been resolved. The perfect healing of tendon tissue requires a sequential and coordinated expression of numerous molecules and GF, each responsible for a specific and distinct process. In the final part of this work, we have taken into consideration the molecules which present themselves as potentially more valid candidates for the activation of the processes of tendon tissue neoformation. Regarding this, it would seem possible that the use of recombining GDFs could be approved for clinical use in the treatment of tendon breakages [103]. Even the Scx would show an applicative interest in this sense, even if it should be used through a gene therapy approach (the most probable of these would seem to be the use of nonviral vectors) since an extracellular application of the protein would not generate any on site effect [103]. However, in this area, further and deeper studies are still necessary which evidence that characterization of the optimal factors adapts to induce the neoformation of tendon tissue in various models of tendon breakage and tendinopathy.

References

1. Leadbetter WB (1995) Anti-inflammatory therapy in sport injury: the role of nonsteroidal drugs and corticosteroid injection. Clin Sports Med 14:353–410
2. Leadbetter WB (1995) Cell-matrix response in tendon injury. Clin Sports Med 14:353–410
3. Bisciotti GN (2010) Le lesioni muscolari. Calzetti e Mariucci (eds). Perugia
4. Józsa LG, Kannus P (1997) Healing and regeneration of tendon. In: Human tendons: anatomy, physiology and pathology. Human Kinetics, Champaign, pp 526–554
5. Holch M, Biewener A, Thermann H, Zwipp H (1994) Non-operative treatment of acute Achilles tendon ruptures: a clinical concept and experimental results. Sport Exerc Injury 1:18–22
6. Maagaard-Mortensen NH, Skov O, Egund N (1994) Regeneration of Achilles tendon after necrosis. Acta Orthop Scand 258(Suppl):65–87
7. Minibattle ZH (1995) Treatment of Achilles tendon rupture. Non operative functional treatment. The second Congress of EFORT, Specialty day of EFFORT. Munich, July 4th 1995. Abstract book p 83
8. Houglum PA (1992) Soft tissue healing and its impact on rehabilitation. J Sport Rehab 1:19–39
9. Józsa LG, Lehto M, Kannus P, Kvist M, Vieno T et al (1989) Fibronectin an laminin in Achilles tendon. Acta Orthop Scand 70:469–471
10. Letho M, Józsa LG, Kvist M, Järvinen M, Bàlint BJ, Rèffy A (1990) Fibronectin in the ruptured human Achilles tendon and its paratenon. An immunoperoxidase study. Ann Chir Gynaecol 79:72–77
11. Enwemeka CS (1989) Inflammation, cellularity, and fibrillogenesis in regenerating tendon: implications for tendon rehabilitation. Phys Ther 69(10):816–825
12. Garret WE, Lohnes J (1990) Cellular and matrix response to mechanical injury at the myotendinous junction. In: Leadbetter WB, Buckwalter JA, Gordon SL (eds) Sport induced inflammation. AAOS, Park Ridge, pp 215–224
13. Okuda Y, Gorski JP, An KN, Amadio PC (1987) Biomechanical, histological and biochemical analyses of canine tendon. J Orthop Res 5:60–68
14. Abrahamsson SO, Lundborg G, Lohmander LS (1989) Segmental variation in microstructure, matrix synthesis and cell proliferation in rabbit flexor tendon. Scand J Plast Reconstr Surg Hand Surg 23(3):191–198

15. Abrahamsson SO, Lundborg G, Lohmander LS (1989) Tendon healing in vivo. An experimental model. Scand J Plast Reconstr Surg Hand Surg 23(3):199–205
16. Dovi JV, He LK, Di Pietro LA (2003) Accelerated wound closure in neutrophil-depleted mice. J Leukoc Biol 73(4):448–455
17. Godbout C, Bilodeau R, Van Rooijen N, Bouchard P, Frenette J (2010) Transient neutropenia increases macrophage accumulation and cell proliferation but does not improve repair following intratendinous rupture of Achilles tendon. J Orthop Res 28(8):1084–1091
18. Mirza R, Di Pietro LA, Koh TJ (2009) Selective and specific macrophage ablation is detrimental to wound healing in mice. Am J Pathol 175(6):2454–2462
19. Khanna S, Biswas S, Shang Y, Collard E, Azad A, Kauh C, Bhasker V, Gordillo GM, Sen CK, Roy S (2010) Macrophage dysfunction impairs resolution of inflammation in the wounds of diabetic mice. PLoS One 5(3):e9539
20. Bréchot N, Gomez E, Bignon M, Khallou-Laschet J, Dussiot M, Cazes A, Alanio-Bréchot C, Durand M, Philippe J, Silvestre JS, Van Rooijen N, Corvol P, Nicoletti A, Chazaud B, Germain S (2008) Modulation of macrophage activation state protects tissue from necrosis during critical limb ischemia in thrombospondin-1-deficient mice. PLoS One 3(12):e3950
21. Hays PL, Kawamura S, Deng XH, Dagher E, Mithoefer K, Ying L, Rodeo SA (2008) The role of macrophages in early healing of a tendon graft in a bone tunnel. J Bone Joint Surg Am 90(3):565–579
22. Sercarz EE, Maverakis E (2004) Recognition and function in a degenerate immune system. Mol Immunol 40(14-15):1003–1008
23. Krysko DV, D'Herde K, Vandenabeele P (2006) Clearance of apoptotic and necrotic cells and its immunological consequences. Apoptosis 11:1709–1726
24. Poon IK, Hulett MD, Parish CR (2010) Molecular mechanism of late apoptotic/necrotic cell clearance. Cell Death Differ 28:340–345
25. Woodall J Jr, Tucci M, Mishra A, Asfour A, Benghuzzi H (2008) Cellular effects of platelet rich plasmainterleukin1 release from prp treated macrophages. Biomed Sci Instrum 44:489–494
26. Andia I, Sanchez M, Maffulli N (2010) Tendon healing and platelet-rich plasma therapies. Expert Opin Biol Ther 10:1–12
27. Scott A, Lian Ø, Roberts CR, Cook JL, Handley CJ, Bahr R, Samiric T, Ilic MZ, Parkinson J, Hart DA, Duronio V, Khan KM (2008) Increased versican content is associated with tendinosis pathology in the patellar tendon of athletes with jumper's knee. Scand J Med Sci Sports 18(4):427–435
28. Scott A, Lian Ø, Bahr R, Hart DA, Duronio V, Khan KM (2008) Increased mast cell numbers in human patellar tendinosis: correlation with symptom duration and vascular hyperplasia. Br J Sports Med 42(9):753–757
29. Del Buono A, Battery L, Denaro V, Maccauro G, Maffulli N (2011) Tendinopathy and inflammation: some truths. Int J Immunopathol Pharmacol 24(1 Suppl 2):45–50
30. Peacock EE, Van Winkle W (1970) Surgery and biology of wound repair. Saunders, Philadelphia, p 331424
31. Katenkamp D, Stiller D, Schulze E (1976) Ultrastructural cytology of regenerating tendon–an experimental study. Exp Pathol (Jena) 12(1):25–37
32. Gelberman RH, Vandeberg JS, Manske PR, Akeson WH (1985) The early stages of flexor tendon healing: a morphologic study of the first fourteen days. J Hand Surg Am 10(6 Pt 1):776–784
33. Gelberman RH, An KA, Banes A, Goldberg V (1988) Tendon. In: Woo S, Buckwalter JA (eds) Injury and repair of the musculoskeletal soft tissue. AAOS, Ark Ridge, pp 1–40
34. Garner WL, McDonald JA, Koo M, Kuhn C 3rd, Weeks PM (1989) Identification of the collagen-producing cells in healing flexor tendons. Plast Reconstr Surg 83(5):875–879
35. Chang J, Most D, Thunder R, Mehrara B, Longaker MT, Lineaweaver WC (1998) Molecular studies in flexor tendon wound healing: the role of basic fibroblast growth factor gene expression. J Hand Surg Am 23:1052–1058

36. Wang JH (2006) Mechanobiology of tendon. J Biomech 39(9):1563–1582
37. Bisciotti GN, Capellu M, Hidalgo J et al (2007) Comparison of stiffness resulting from different surgical methods of repair of Achilles tendon rupture. Min Ort Traum 58(2):107–114
38. Everts V, Van der Zee E, Creemers L, Beertsen W (1996) Phagocytosis and intracellular digestion of collagen, its role in turnover and remodeling. Histochem J 28:229–245
39. Ackermann PW, Ahmed M, Kreicbergs A (2002) Early nerve regeneration after Achilles tendon rupture – a prerequisite for healing? A study in the rat. J Orthop Res 20:849–856
40. Stayaert AE, Burssens PJ, Vercruysse CW et al (2006) The effects of substance P on the biomechanics properties of ruptured rat Achilles' tendon. Arch Phys Med Rehabil 87:254–258
41. Burssens P, Stayaert A, Forsyth R et al (2005) Exogenously administered substance P and neutral endopeptidase inhibitors stimulate fibroblast proliferation, angiogenesis, and collagen organization during Achilles tendon healing. Foot Ankle Int 26:832–839
42. Carlsson O, Schizas N, Li J, Ackermann PW (2011) Substance P injections enhance tissue proliferation and regulate sensory nerve ingrowth in rat tendon repair. Scand J Med Sci Sports 21(4):562–569
43. Mammoto T, Seerattan RA, Paulson KD et al (2008) Nerve growth factor improves ligament healing. J Orthop Res 26:957–964
44. Ivie TJ, Bray RC, Salo PT (2002) Denervation impairs healing of the rabbit medial collateral ligament. J Orthop Res 20:990–995
45. Nelson L, Fairclough J, Archer CW (2010) Use of stem cells in the biological repair of articular cartilage. Expert Opin Biol Ther 10:43–55
46. Lui PP, Cheuk YC, Hung LK, Fu CF (2007) Increased apoptosis at the late stage of tendon healing. Wound Repair Regen 15:702–707
47. Hengartner MO (2000) The biochemistry of apoptosis. Nature 407:770–776
48. Kaufmann SH, Hengartner MO (2001) Programmed cell death: alive and well in the new millennium. Trends Cell Biol 11:526–534
49. Barkhausen T, Van Griensven M, Zeichen J, Bosch U (2003) Modulation of cell function of human tendon fibroblast by different repetitive cyclic mechanical stress patterns. Exp Toxicol Pathol 55:153–158
50. Stutek M, Van Griensven M, Zeichen J, Brauer N, Bosch U (2003) Cyclic mechanical stretching of human patellar tendon fibroblast: activation of JNK and modulation of apoptosis. Knee Surg Sports Traumatol Arthrosc 11:122–129
51. Scott A, Khan KM, Herr J, Cook JL, Lian O, Duronio V (2005) Hight strain mechanical loading rapidly induces tendon apoptosis: an ex vivo rat tibialis anterior model. Br J Sports Med 39:25
52. Blumenthal NC, Ricci C, Breger L, Zychlinsky A, Solomon H et al (1997) Effects of low-intensity AC and/or DC electromagnetic fields on cell attachment and induction of apoptosis. Biolectromagnetics 18:264–272
53. Yuan J, Murrel GA, Trickett A, Wang MX (2003) Involvement of cytochrome c release and caspase-3 activation in the oxidative stress-induced apoptosis in human tendon fibroblast. Biochim Biophys Acta 1641:35–41
54. Sendzik J, Shakibaei M, Schafer-Korting M, Stahlmann R (2005) Fluoroquinolones cause changes in extracellular matrix, signaling proteins, metalloproteinases and caspase-3 in cultured human tendon cells. Toxicology 212:24–36
55. Hosaka Y, Teraoka H, Yamamoto E, Ueda H, Takehana K (2005) Mechanism of cell death in inflamed superficial digital flexor tendon in horse. J Comp Pathol 132:51–58
56. Chuen FS, Chuk CY, Ping WY, Nar WW, Kim HL, Ming CK (2004) Immunohistochemical characterization of cells in adult human patellar tendon. J Histochem Cytochem 52:1151–1157
57. Daugas E, Nochy D, Ravagnag L, Loeffer M et al (2000) Apoptosis-inducing factor (AIF): a ubiquitous mitochondrial oxidoreductase involved in apoptosis. FEBS Lett 476:118–123

58. Desmouliere A (1995) Factors influencing myofibroblast differentiation during wound healing and fibrosis. Cell Biol Int 19:471–476
59. Gabbiani G (2003) The myofibroblast in wound healing and fibrocontractive disease. J Pathol 200(4):500–503
60. Kuroda R, Kurosaka M, Yoshiya S, Mizuno K (2000) Localization of growth factors in the reconstructed anterior cruciate ligament: immunohistological study in dogs. Knee Surg Sports Traumatol Arthrosc 8:120–126
61. Visser LC, Arnoczky SP, Caballero O, Egerbacher M (2010) Platelet-rich fibrin constructs elute higher concentrations of transforming growth factor-β1 and increase tendon cell proliferation over time when compared to blood clots: a comparative in vitro analysis. Vet Surg 39(7):811–817
62. Duffy FJ Jr, Seiler JG, Gelberman RH, Hergrueter CA (1995) Growth factors and canine flexor tendon healing: initial studies in uninjured and repair models. J Hand Surg Am 20:645–649
63. Chang J, Most D, Stelnicki E, Siebert JW, Longaker MT, Hui K, Lineaweaver WC (1997) Gene expression of transforming growth factor beta-1 in rabbit zone II flexor tendon wound healing: evidence for dual mechanisms of repair. Plast Reconstr Surg 100:937–944
64. Oryan A, Moshiri A (2011) A long term study on the role of exogenous human recombinant basic fibroblast growth factor on the superficial digital flexor tendon healing in rabbits. J Musculoskelet Neuronal Interact 11(2):185–189
65. Bidder M, Towler DA, Gelberman RH, Boyer MI (2000) Expression of mRNA for vascular endothelial growth factor at the repair site of healing canine flexor tendon. J Orthop Res 18:247–252
66. Savitskaya YA, Izaguirre A, Sierra L, Perez F, Cruz F, Villalobos E, Almazan A, Ibarra C (2011) Effect of angiogenesis-related cytokines on rotator cuff disease: the search for sensitive biomarkers of early tendon degeneration. Clin Med Insights Arthritis Musculoskelet Disord 4:43–53
67. Chang SC (1994) Cartilage-derived morphogenetic proteins. J Biol Chem 269:28227–28234
68. Tsubone T, Moran SL, Amadio PC, Zhao C, An KN (2004) Expression of growth factors in canine flexor tendon after laceration in vivo. Ann Plast Surg 53(4):393–397
69. Chen CH, Cao Y, Wu YF, Bais AJ, Gao JS, Tang JB (2008) Tendon healing in vivo: gene expression and production of multiple growth factors in early tendon healing period. J Hand Surg Am 33(10):1834–1842
70. Potenza AD (1962) Tendon healing within the flexor digital sheath in the dog: an experimental study. J Bone Joint Surg Am 44:49–64
71. Bergljung L (1968) Vascular reactions after tendon suture and tendon transplantation. A stereo-microangiographic study on the calcaneal tendon of the rabbit. Scand J Plast Reconstr Surg Suppl 4:7–63
72. Takasugi H, Inoue H, Akahori O (1976) Scanning electron microscopy of repaired tendon and pseudosheat. Hand 8:228–234
73. Matthews P (1979) The pathology of flexor tendon repair. Hand 11:233–242
74. Mass DP, Tuel RJ (1991) Intrinsic healing of the laceration site in human superficialis flexor tendons in vitro. J Hand Surg Am 16(1):24–30
75. Williams IF, Heaton A, McCullagh KG (1980) Cell morphology and collagen types in equine tendon scar. Res Vet Sci 28(3):302–310
76. Schneider LH (1987) Flexor tenolysis. In: Hunter JM, Schneider LH, Mackin EJ (eds) Tendon surgery in the hand. Mosby, St Louis, pp 209–215
77. Wheeldon T (1939) The use of cellophane as a permanent tendon sheat. J Bone Joint Surg 21:393–405
78. Lundborg G (1976) Experimental flexor tendon healing without adhesion formation – A new concept of tendon nutrition and intrinsic healing mechanism. Hand 8:235–238

79. Lundborg G, Hansson HA, Rank F, Rydevik B (1980) Superficial repair of severed flexor tendon in synovial environment. An experimental ultrastructural study on cellular mechanism. J Hand Surg Am 5:451–461
80. Manske PE, Gelberman RH, Vandeberg JS, Lesker AP (1984) Intrinsic flexor-tendon repair. A morphologic study in vivo. J Bone Joint Surg Am 66:385–396
81. Lindsay WK, Thomson HG (1960) Digital flexor tendons: an experimental study. Part I. The significance of each component of the flexor mechanism in tendon healing. Br J Plast Surg 12:289–316
82. Gelberman RH, Vandeberg JS, Manske PR, Akesn WH (1983) Flexor tendon healing and restoration of the gliding surface. An ultrastructural study in dogs. J Bone Joint Surg Am 65:70–80
83. Lundborg G, Rank F (1987) Tendon healing: intrinsic mechanism. In: Hunter JM, Schneider LH, Mackin EJ (eds) Tendon surgery in the hand. Mosby, St. Louis, pp 54–60
84. Fenwick SA, Hazleman BL, Riley GP (2002) The vasculature and its role in the damaged and healing tendon. Arthritis Res 4(4):252–260
85. Aspenberg P (2007) Stimulation of tendon repair: mechanical loading, GDFs and platelets. A minireview. Int Orthop 31:783–789
86. Herpin A, Lelong C, Favrel P (2004) Transforming growth factor-beta-related proteins: an ancestral and widespread superfamily of cytokines in metazoans. Dev Comp Immunol 28:461–485
87. Storm EE, Huynh TV, Copeland NG, Jenkins NA, Kingsley DM, Lee SJ (1994) Limb alterations in brachypodism mice due to mutations in a new member of the TGF-b superfamily. Nature 368:639–642
88. Storm E, Kingsley DM (1996) Joint patterning defects caused by single and double mutations in members of the bone morphogenetic protein (BMP) family. Development 122:3969–3979
89. Mikic B (2004) Multiple effects of GDF-5 deficiency on skeletal tissues: implications for therapeutic bioengineering. Ann Biomed Eng 32:466–476
90. Harada M et al (2007) Developmental failure of the intra-articular ligaments in mice with absence of growth differentiation factor 5. Osteoarthritis Cartilage 15:468–474
91. Wolfman NM et al (1997) Ectopic induction of tendon and ligament in rats by growth and differentiation factors 5, 6, and 7, members of the TGFbeta gene family. J Clin Invest 100:321–330
92. Dines JS et al (2007) The effect of growth differentiation factor-5-coated sutures on tendon repair in a rat model. J Shoulder Elbow Surg 16:S204–S207
93. Aspenberg P, Forslund C (1999) Enhanced tendon healing with GDF 5 and 6. Acta Orthop Scand 70:51–54
94. Rickert M et al (2005) Adenovirus-mediated gene transfer of growth and differentiation factor-5 into tenocytes and the healing rat Achilles tendon. Connect Tissue Res 46:175–183
95. Hotten GC et al (1996) Recombinant human growth/differentiation factor 5 stimulates mesenchyme aggregation and chondrogenesis responsible for the skeletal development of limbs. Growth Factors 13:65–74
96. Kakudo N, Wang YB, Miyake S, Kushida S, Kusumoto K (2007) Analysis of osteochondro-induction using growth and differentiation factor-5 in rat muscle. Life Sci 81:137–143
97. Kadesch T (1993) Consequences of heteromeric interactions among helix-loop-helix proteins. Cell Growth Differ 4:49–55
98. Murre C et al (1989) Interactions between heterologous helix-loop-helix proteins generate complexes that bind specifically to a common DNA sequence. Cell 58:537–544
99. Brent AE, Schweitzer R, Tabin CJ (2003) A somitic compartment of tendon progenitors. Cell 113:235–248
100. Cserjesi P, Brown D, Ligon KL, Lyons GE, Copeland NG, Gilbert DJ, Jenkins NA, Olson EN (1995) Scleraxis: a basic helix-loop-helix protein that prefigures skeletal formation during mouse embryogenesis. Development 121:1099–1110

101. Léjard V (2007) Scleraxis and NFATc regulate the expression of the pro-alpha1(I) collagen gene in tendon fibroblasts. J Biol Chem 282:17665–17675
102. Murchison N et al (2007) Regulation of tendon differentiation by scleraxis distinguishes force-transmitting tendons from muscle-anchoring tendons. Development 134:2697–2708
103. Aslan H, Kimelman-Bleich N, Pelled G, Gazit D (2008) Molecular targets for tendon neoformation. J Clin Invest 118(2):439–444

Chapter 3
Adductor Tendinopathy

Jean-Marcel Ferret, Yannick Barthélémy, and Matthieu Lechauve

Abstract Adductor pain is very common in sports, but it is essential to distinguish among true tendinopathy, which is an enthesopathy (adductor longus insertion pain on the pubis), a tear of the myotendinous junction, which is rarer, and projected pain, where the adductors are affected the victims rather than being the cause: in abdominal groin pain (pubalgia) and all hip problems, especially femoral acetabular impingement (FAI), which affects young athletic population. Adductor tendinopathy can be isolated, but is also often associated with pubalgia. Once a positive diagnosis has been established, treatment can be tailored to the cause: medical for isolated tendinopathy, and often surgical in the form associated with pubalgia. Abdominal parietal pain is often the evolution of neglected adductor tendinopathy, which is why we must encourage those in the sporting environment to be more rigorous in the management of this pathological condition.

3.1 Introduction

Adductor pain is very common in sport, especially in activities with acceleration, deceleration, sudden changes in direction, blocking, trunk rotation, sliding tackles, and kicking: football, rugby, handball, and ice hockey [1, 2]. According to different authors, the epidemiology of adductor pain varies from 5 [2] to 16% of all injuries in soccer players [3, 4].

J.-M. Ferret (✉)
Sporea Lyon, 3 rue Pierre Corneille, Lyon 69006, France
e-mail: jmfemslc@orange.fr

Y. Barthélémy
Charleroi Sport Santé, Rue de Goutroux, 39. 6031, Monceau Sur Sambre, Belgium
e-mail: yannick.barthelemy78@gmail.com; yannick.barthelemy@chu-charleroi.be

M. Lechauve
Clinic of Al Hilal Saudi FC, Riyad, Kingdom of Saudi Arabia
e-mail: matthieulechauve@hotmail.fr

G.N. Bisciotti, P. Volpi (eds.), *The Lower Limb Tendinopathies*,
Sports and Traumatology, DOI 10.1007/978-3-319-33234-5_3

Adductor tendinopathy corresponds to one of the four forms of sport groin pain:

- Abdominal parietal failure
- Pubis arthropathy
- Enthesopathy adductors
- Enthesopathy rectus abdominis

These pathological conditions do indeed have a common location, all around the symphysis pubis, which plays the role of a true anatomical and functional crossroads. They occur within a common framework, consisting of mechanical stress to the pubic region, due to the practice of sports. Moreover, these four pathological conditions are often intertwined in athletes, although they can occur in isolation. The tendinopathy physiopathology is a multifactorial process, involving intrinsic and extrinsic factors that evolve independently or in combination [5]. In particular, repetitive mechanical loads and/or the application of loads exceeding the strength of the tendon may gradually cause microscopic and macroscopic lesions. Collagen fibers start to denature, gradually causing tendinitis [6].

3.2 Anatomy

3.2.1 Adductor Muscle

The adductor muscles (longus, brevis, magnus, pectineus, and gracilis) have a proximal insertion into the subpubic area with the internal obturator. The pectineus lies above and beyond the pubic tubercle, along the pubic crest. The gracilis originates inside the adductor on the front of the pubis and internal third of the lower edge of ischiopubic branch (Fig. 3.1).

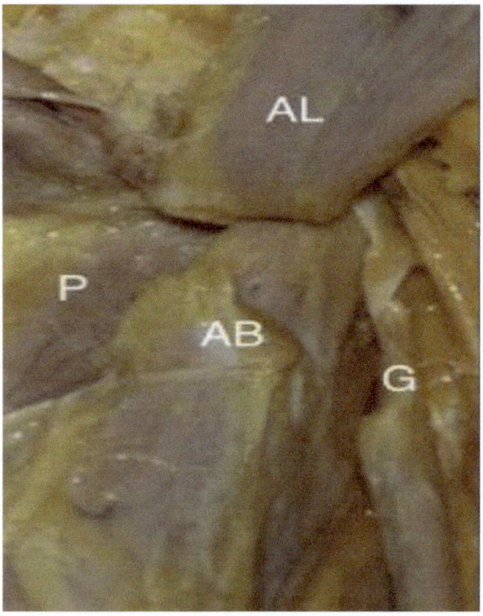

Fig. 3.1 Cadaveric adductor anatomy (Pesquer collection)

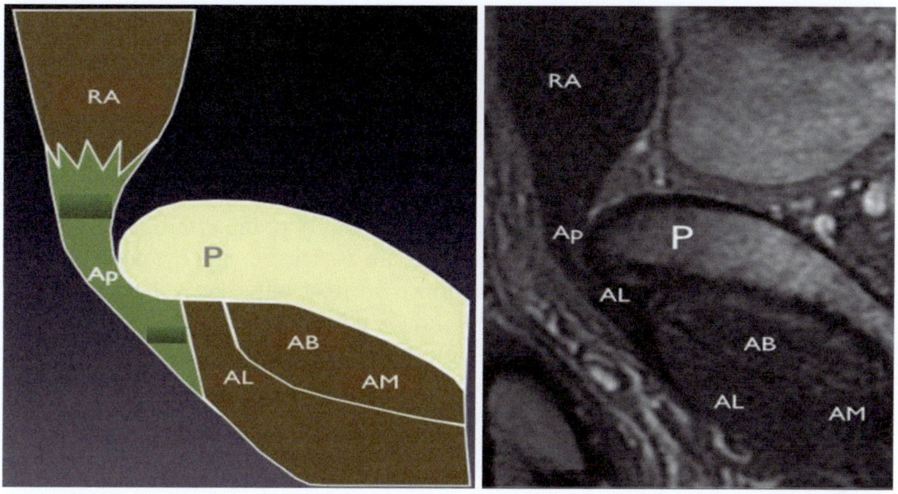

Fig. 3.2 Adductor anatomy on MRI (Pesquer Collection)

The proximal insertion of the adductor longus is close to the pubic tubercle and pubic symphysis through the tendon fibers (40 %) in area and the muscle fibers (60 %) in depth. Brevis and magnus adductor insertion is only muscular [7, 8]. The adductor longus tendon is small, measuring 11.6 mm long and 3.7 mm wide, according to a cadaver study [9]. It is the only adductor, to have an individualized tendon. There is an anatomical continuum through a common fascia between the surface fibers of the adductor longus tendon and the distal tendon of the rectus abdominis. This fascia is in contact with the fibrocartilaginous disk of the pubic symphysis and the capsular structures. These anatomical data explain why painful irradiation of one or more of the affected structures can extend to the thigh and the abdomen (Fig. 3.2) [10].

3.2.2 *Inguinal Region*

The inguinal region is located in the lower part of the abdomen, delimited by the outer edge of the rectus abdominis inside, by the oblique and transverse abdominal muscles outside, by the inguinal ligament at the bottom, and by the oblique internal and transverse muscles at the top. The inguinal canal lies between the muscle layers. The anterior inguinal wall consists of the external oblique fascia; the fibers diverge to create the superficial inguinal ring. The space between the inguinal ligament at the bottom and the conjoint tendon at the top is closed by the transverse fascia. It is a thin and solid membrane that is in contact with the peritoneum. The outer part of this area is the deep inguinal orifice, through which spermatic cord components pass to the testis. The peritoneum is located behind the transverse fascia plane. The iliohypogastric, ilioinguinal, and genitofemoral nerves pass behind the external oblique fascia, in front of the muscles.

3.3 Definition and Differential Diagnosis

The type of complaint is not unequivocal: we immediately eliminate acute pathological conditions, such as bone avulsion of the pubis and a myotendinous tear of the adductor. Moreover, distinction should be made between true adductor tendinopathy, i.e., insertional tendinopathy or enthesopathy [7, 11], and pain of locoregional origin such as groin pain due to abdominal injury or hip arthropathy. Indeed, in this case, different pathological conditions are associated, and the adductors are the victims rather than the cause. Our aim is to treat only the isolated adductor enthesopathy. Adductor enthesopathy essentially concerns the adductor longus with a prevalence of 45–60 % [12]. First, we must eliminate all pathological conditions with groin pain that is not caused by adductor longus enthesopathy and especially abdominal groin pain and hip arthropathy [13].

3.3.1 Abdominal Groin Pain

In the case of abdominal groin pain, the pathological condition may start with a mild pain of the adductor, which is often neglected, but can quickly become complicated abdominal wall pain with an unpredictable evolution. Clinical examination of the abdominal wall is aimed at helping to refine the diagnosis: rectus abdominis tendinitis, pathological condition of the inguinal ring and abdominal wall (athletic pubalgia), inguinal hernia, tunnel syndromes, and obturator, iliohypogastric, ilioinguinal, and symphysis arthropathy [14].

Questioning together with clinical and complementary examination (imaging, EMG) easily eliminate rectus abdominis tendinitis, symphysis arthropathy, inguinal hernia, and tunnel syndromes. Examination of the inguinal canal is imperative in the context of long adductor tendinopathy. The deep inguinal ring, including failure of the transverse fascia, would then be involved. In the chronic form, the painful symptoms are often exacerbated by the increased abdominal pressure.

For athletic pubalgia, the primary functional sign is inguinal pain with coughing, especially after effort, and abdominal pain when athletes sit up in bed after waking up. External orifice and deep orifice palpation must be bilateral and comparative information on a patient standing, the scrotum is pumped and forefinger palpates the channel up, out, and back. A Valsalva maneuver helps to inform the test. Clinical examination finds an enlarged inguinal ring, and an impulsive and painful cough. This form, if it does not show improvement after 2 months of well-conducted rehabilitation work, requires a surgical opinion [15]. The disorder differs from a real inguinal hernia in that only one protrusion or bulging fascia was found during Valsalva maneuvers [16]. Adductor tendinopathy, in this context, is an associated pathological condition.

The treatment is adapted to the pathological condition, which requires a very precise diagnosis because there are numerous intricate forms. Early diagnosis is essential for rehabilitation treatment to be efficient. Surgery has its place in forms resistant to medical treatment, particularly in cases of inguinal canal posterior wall deficiency [14, 17].

In professional clubs, individual screening for athletes at risk should be systematic early in the season and preventive care should be performed throughout the season.

3.3.2 Hip

Hip pain is the other essential diagnosis. Indeed, any abnormality of the hip can cause adductor pain. This phenomenon is well known for hip osteoarthritis, but less so in femoral acetabular impingement (FAI) [18, 19]. When diagnosing any adductor pain that is resistant to treatment, a hip problem must be eliminated [20, 21]. This will be systematically reviewed and any limitation of the range of motion (ROM) taken into consideration. In FAI, a pathognomonic sign is pain on hip flexion, adduction, and internal rotation (FADIR: Fig. 3.3). Another important sign is pain, after effort, on hip flexion (for example, in our experience, pain after a soccer game when a player uses his hip in flexion >90° braking or acceleration), a sign never found in abdominal groin pain. FAI concerns physical activities with ballistic hip movements of large amplitude, such as soccer, martial arts, and artistic dance [18].

Characteristics of FAI are:

- Cam lesion: additional bone seen, more frequently at the antero-superior position of the femoral head neck junction [22, 23]; it is the most frequent lesion in soccer [24].
- Pincer impingement of the hip due to a change in the acetabulum: deep or retroverted acetabulum [29].
- A combination of the two.

The premature contact of the head–neck junction of the hip with the acetabulum caused by a cam or pincer bony abnormality causes pain in the inguinal area for activities with flexion, adduction, and medial rotation [25].

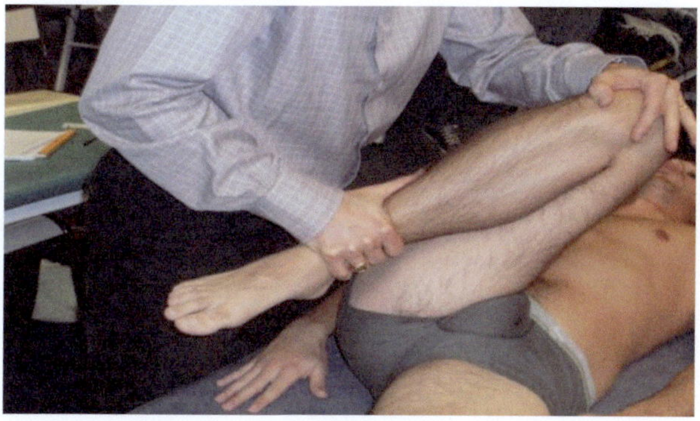

Fig. 3.3 Pain in flexion, adduction, internal rotation (FADIR) of the hip

High-level activities in childhood give rise to the risk of cam-type deformity [26], possibly in relation to a minimally slipped capital femoral epiphysis [27].

Imaging is important for evaluating FAI: to define the type of lesions and to adapt therapy. Plain X-rays and contrast-enhanced MRI are sufficient.

Rest or decreased activity: avoidance of hip hyperflexion, associated with hip rehabilitation therapy (on a bicycle with no resistance, 100 turns per minute for 20 min daily), lumbar and gluteal muscle strengthening, and postural work are sufficient, in most of cases, to enable a return to sport. However, in some cases, surgery may be needed (arthroscopy, mini-arthrotomy [28, 29].

Other pathological conditions of the hip to eliminate by rigorous clinical examination and imaging are:

- Coxarthropathy
- Acetabular labral tear
- Slipped capital femoral epiphysis (childhood pathological condition)
- Femoral head osteonecrosis
- Femoral neck and ischiopubic branch stress fracture
- Osteochondrosis or avulsion of the antero-inferior iliac spine (adolescent pathological condition)

3.3.3 Other Differential Diagnoses

- Hip muscle injury: iliopsoas, lateral and medial rotator, and iliopsoas bursitis
- Radicular syndrome: obturator neuralgia
- Inflammatory rheumatism: rheumatoid polyarthritis and ankylosing spondylarthritis
- Infectious lesions: symphysis osteitis
- Metabolic arthropathy: hyperuricemia
- Benign tumors: osteoid osteoma; malignant tumors, osteosarcoma

3.4 Etiopathogenesis

This intimate relationship among the adductor longus, the rectus abdominis, and the pubic symphysis is the anatomical substrate of biomechanical assembly to ensure the stability of the anterior pelvis and transmission of forces from both sides of the pubis [7]. This “confluence” of anatomical elements explains the frequency of associated damage among the different clinical forms [30]. Pesquer et al., in a retrospective series of 180 patients operated on to treat adductor tendinopathy, found that 80 % of patients had associated parietal failure requiring surgical treatment [31].

There are two types of risk factors for adductor tendinopathy.

3.4.1 Intrinsic Factors

The pathogenesis of tendinopathy adductor insertion is related to functional overload and repetitive strain injuries caused by twisting and pulling tendon insertions [32, 33]. In particular, some sports predispose to groin pain, such as soccer, Australian and American football, and ice hockey.

Soccer player morphotype characterized by association of a lack of extensibility of the anterior and posterior chains, hyperlordosis with pelvic anteversion, and genu varum and flexum of the knee, causes an overload of the adductor. The analysis of the morphological type of an athlete is important. The examination of the spine and lumbopelvic hinge assesses the overall static equilibrium of the patient's pelvis and the joint mobility of the different segments. A pelvic tilt due to legs of unequal length can be corrected if necessary. Anteversion of the pelvis is also reported to be a risk factor for groin pain [19, 37]. The use of a biplanar imaging system with a low X-ray dose (EOS) seems promising in the overall systematic analysis of the static lumbar–pelvic complex.

Many authors believe that the origin of the pain is due to a muscle imbalance in stabilizing the pelvis between the strong and retracted adductors and a weak abdominal wall [34, 35]; other authors describe an imbalance of the hip adductor and abductors as a cause of groin pain [36].

Any limitation in the ROM of the hip causes an adductor malfunction. Soccer is the best example because at 20 years old, professional players have a significant limitation of flexion (8 %), abduction (30 %), and adduction (35 %) in comparison with the general population of the same age [38].

The ballistic movements of large amplitude inflict significant pressures and microtraumas upon the femoroacetabular joint, notably during shooting with to arm it: hip extension, abduction, lateral rotation, and at the end of movement flexion, adduction, and medial rotation [18]. This could explain the limitations in amplitude in the young professional player (Figs. 3.4 and 3.5).

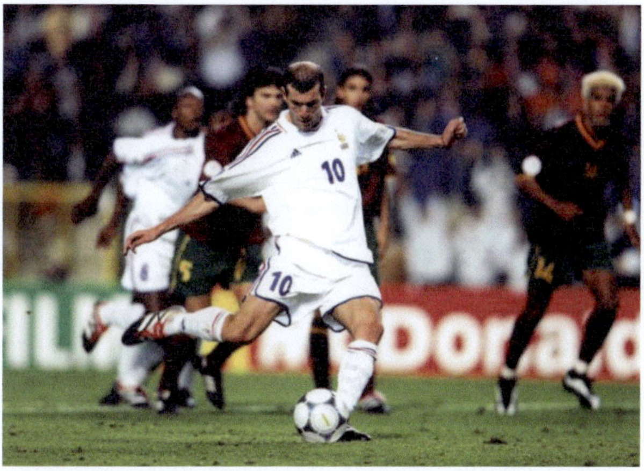

Fig. 3.4 Beggining of shooting movement: extension, abduction and lateral rotation of the hip, knee flexion

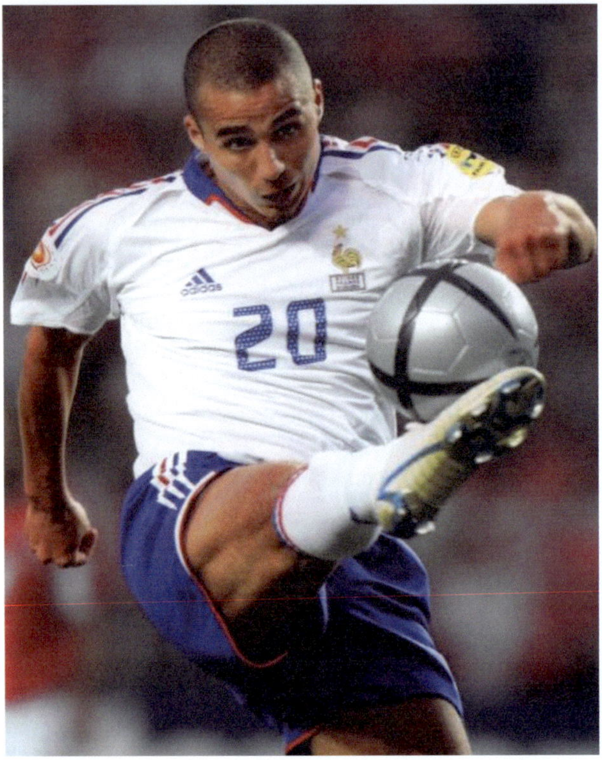

Fig. 3.5 End of shoot movement

Flexion, adduction, and medial rotation of the hip, and knee extension:

- The succession of accelerations, blockages, direction changes, rotations, jump receptions, and striking involve so much pressure being exercised all over the lumbar–pelvic–femoral complex, explaining the hyperuse of adductors and the abdominal wall. The abdominal cavity consists mainly of water and therefore is slightly compressible. Any work done without abdominal sheathing and pelvic retroversion increases abdominal pressure with a push on the anterior abdominal wall. Repeated abdominal strengthening exercises in a bad position, e.g, pelvis anteversion or hyperlordosis, contribute to abdominal wall distension, in addition to the practice of sports involving rotation and pivoting that exert considerable force on the lumbar–pelvic–femoral complex with increased abdominal pressure [39].

Other Etiologies

- Static troubles of the lower extremity: inequality, static disorders of the feet.
- Hygienic or dietary problems:
  - Lack of hydration
  - Acidifying diet: food too rich in sugars and animal proteins
  - Poor dental status promoting chronic inflammation

3.4.2 *Extrinsic Factors*

Extrinsic factors that are involved in this overuse at groin, particularly:

- Ground quality: hard ground, for example, road training, frozen ground, soggy pitch
- Atmospheric conditions: wind and rain
- Change of playing surface: grass, synthetic or canvas shoes, crampons
- Excessive physical activity, a sudden increase in training load, loss of fitness after injury
- Bad programming of training, inappropriate content, disorganized competition schedule, overpressure of abdominal work

3.5 Clinic

Precise questioning must precede the clinical examination: pain severity (diagnostic consultation is often late), pain location at the root of the thigh, sudden appearance or gradual, irradiation of the medial face of thigh, pain on effort or after effort, no pain when coughing, no pain when the subject sits up in bed upon waking or in hip flexion (sitting or driving) [18]. The clinical examination should be performed at rest and after effort, which increases symptoms and enables a more accurate diagnosis and prediction of evolution. In the case of adductor tendinopathy, examination is characterized by adductor insertion pain; it radiates into the medial face of the thigh with adductors more or less painfully and contracting.

Its intensity is variable, it may:

- Prevent sports activity
- Cause only gene decreasing sports performance
- Cause annoyance in daily life
- Rest has a favorable influence; sleep is usually not disturbed, but possibility of adductor mornig stiffness.

The main symptom is pain on palpation of the adductor longus insertion on the pubis, this being the only adductor with an individualized tendon; indeed, other adductors fit directly to the bone owing to their muscle fibers [8, 31].

Two other signs confirm the diagnosis:

Pain on adductor stretching due to hip abduction, knee in flexion (FABER; Fig. 3.6)
Pain on resisted adduction from the same position, but also:

- Absence or mild soreness when resisting contraction of hip flexors; indeed, adductors are hip flexor accessories
- Absence of pain on abdominal wall palpation: rectus abdominis pubis insertion, symphysis, inguinal ring
- Absence of pain on trunk flexor when resisting contraction
- No pain when coughing
  It should be noted that in many cases, the clinical form is associated, and it is not rare to find positive tests for several anatomical entities. The tests used must be as sensitive, specific, and reproducible as possible [40].

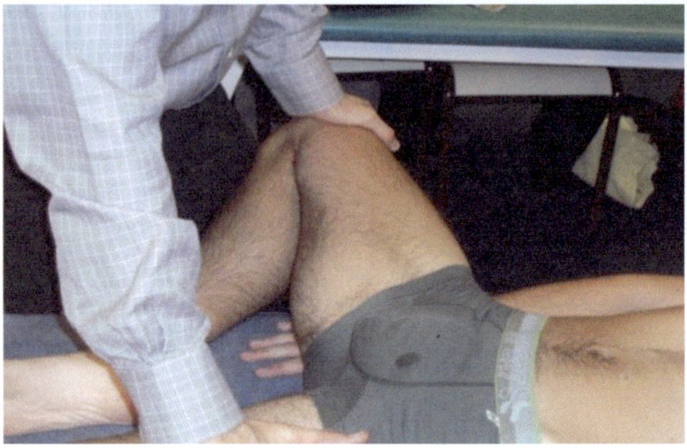

Fig. 3.6 Flexion abduction external rotation (FABER) movement

3.5.1 Biology

Any abnormality must move towards another diagnosis.

3.5.2 Evolution

The evolution is unpredictable from the start: rapid healing or chronicity. Recurrence is very common: 26 % in a population of athletes followed for up to 22 months for a pathological condition of the adductor longus [41].

3.6 Imaging

3.6.1 X-Ray

Adductor longus tendinopathy diagnosis is based on ultrasound and MRI, but standard X-rays are essential for studying the bone matrix, the pubic symphysis, the femoral hip, and pelvic imbalance. Standard radiography with the patient in a balancing on one leg also demonstrates the instability of the pelvis. Instability is discussed when there is a mismatch of ischiopubic branches of 2- or 7-mm diastasis [42].

3.6.2 MRI

Adductor longus tendinopathy manifested as peripheral and central T2 signal enhancement without fluid character and enhancement after gadolinium injection is associated with morphological abnormalities (thickening of the tendon, fissure or avulsion) [31, 44]. These discrepancies, notably T2 signal enhancement, are still

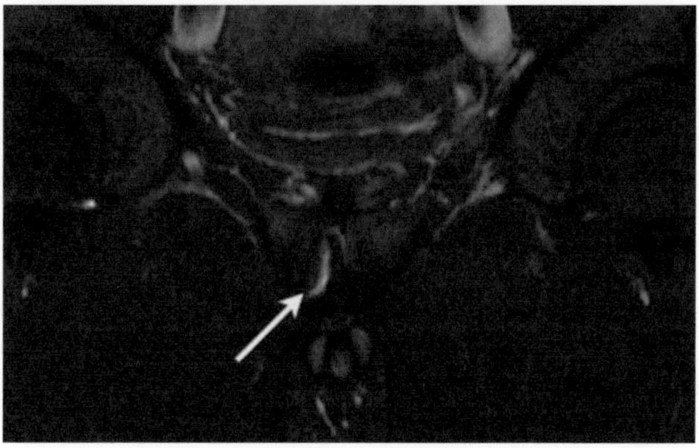

Fig. 3.7 Secondary cleft (Pesquer collection)

inconsistent in the absence of a fissure, recent bleeding or avulsion. This could be explained by the frequency of fibrotic lesions, calcifications and microcalcifications found intraoperatively and pathologically. One study showed that intratendinous abnormalities are sometimes minimal or absent on MRI and edema of the trabecular bone of anterior inferior topography is the only evidence of impairment of the aponeurosis (proven by surgery). The monitoring over time of these anomalies also shows that there is a progression of lesions to a typical aspect of a “secondary cleft” (Fig. 3.7) [10]. The secondary cleft corresponds to an extension of the lesion of the common fascia deep to the capsule down to the groin and in continuity with the primary physiological cleft [10, 31].

There is a strong correlation among the side of the pain, the presence of the sign, and the abnormalities found on MRI and symphysis pubic arthrography [43].

3.6.3 Echography

Ultrasound is widely used because of its ready availability and the spatial resolution allowed by the latest generation of hardware. It is performed with the patient lying down, the hip in flexion, abduction, and external rotation, using a linear high frequency transducer [31, 46]. The adductor analysis is guided clinically by identifying the protrusion of the adductor longus to the anteromedial side of the thigh. Longitudinal and axial slices are usually made and mandatorily compared with the contralateral side.

In sports, asymptomatic microcalcifications are often associated with cortical irregularities, which reflect an old enthesopathy. It is important to analyze the superficial side of the adductor longus tendon: it appears, in healthy subjects, regular and irregular, associated with ulcers of tendinopathy [31, 44]. If enthesopathy is recent or not, it is difficult to distinguish with certainty, and hyperemia can be recognized on color Doppler, but remains an inconstant sign. At a more advanced stage, the tendon is hypertrophic and there are often fissures, which may be longitudinal or transverse. These are more common and correspond to the secondary cleft described on MRI [45].

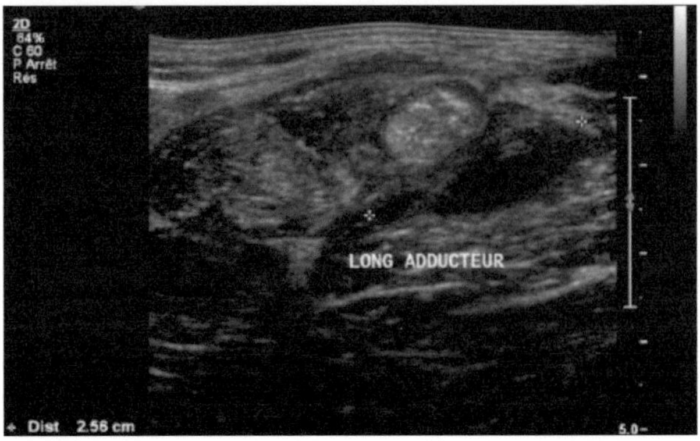

Fig. 3.8 Adductor longus disinsertion (Ph. Tanji collection)

In cases of acute pathological conditions, disinsertion may be asserted if the muscle belly of the adductor longus is significantly retracted, i.e., more than 2 cm from the bone insertion and if there is hematic fluid collection (Fig. 3.8).

Finally, ultrasound study, thanks to its dynamic specificity, is useful for looking for signs of parietal weakness in the superficial inguinal ring. In athletes, we do not expect to see a hernia sac to surface through the inguinal canal, but rather a bulging medial side (direct hernia) or lateral side (indirect hernia) of the caudal epigastric artery during the Valsalva maneuver [19]. This bulge is often symmetrical. There are a significant number of false-positives with impressive bulges but without groin pain. Ultrasound is thwarted in this diagnosis of sports hernia, which remains mainly a clinical diagnosis and may be the cause of long adductor tendinopathy [46].

3.7 Treatment

3.7.1 Conservative Treatment

3.7.1.1 Medical

Early diagnosis and management are crucial. Any adductor pain, even minor, must be supported with a rigorous full clinical examination to clarify the diagnosis and management, but in any case a few days' (5–7) rest is essential, combined with physiotherapy and mechanical treatments: stretching, slow speed eccentric load, and, optionally, NSAIDs. In our experience in professional soccer, this course of action is often sufficient to avoid complications and chronicity. The mistake not to make is to let the player continue with training and matches while on NSAIDs, because under these conditions the transition to chronicity is almost inevitable.

In chronic forms, treatment will be the same, but for a much longer period, emphasizing the eccentric loads at slow speed not only on the adductors, but also on abdominal wall and hip flexors owing to the entanglement of the anatomical structures. We believe that an isokinetic dynamometer is an indispensable tool for this type of treatment.

Oral administration of NSAIDs can be a useful adjuvant treatment. However, the corticosteroid injections should be avoided because of the risk of collagen disorganization and tendon rupture. They should be progressively replaced by PRP (platelet-rich plasma, plasma rich in growth factors [PRGF]) [74] techniques, whose results are notable as they are associated with the eccentric working protocol at a low speed on an isokinetic dynamometer [71].

3.7.2 *Rehabilitation Protocol*

The results of nonsurgical management are based on commitment to the proposed treatment by the athlete and long-term compliance. Rehabilitation is carried out in stages, with close medical supervision. The duration of a level depends on the ability of the athlete to perform the exercises without pain.

It has been proven several times that the use of active programs (unlike the passive physiotherapy) decreases recovery time and return to the game, produces the best long-term results and decreases the risk of recurrence. In particular, mention is made of interesting results (level 1 evidence) through programs combining flexibility exercises, in particular, adductor strengthening and/or abdominal muscles [19, 47].

The first randomized study showed a return to sport 7 months after the beginning of the treatment, to the previous level without pain, in 79 % of the athletes of the group that undertook "active exercises", compared with only 14 % in the group that had "passive physiotherapy" [48].

The rehabilitation program is codified into four stages, which vary in length from 8 to 12 weeks.

3.7.2.1 The First Phase

The goal of the first phase is pain reduction and the elimination of triggers. At least a relative rest from sports of varying duration is essential, in addition to strict refrain from movements that trigger pain.

The practitioner begins his work by normalizing muscle tension (osteopathy, contracting–released stretching, myotension and myofascial work) in painful areas, but also working remotely on pelvic balance, particularly the psoas. It continues with work on mobility of the hip and spine, Cyriax deep transverse massage (DTM) or administration of extracorporeal shock waves to the affected entheses.

From the 3rd day, the practice of manual eccentric loads to the adductor gradually improves tendon resistance by resisted adduction and hip flexion (adductors are accessory hip flexors). Owing to the entanglement of the anatomical structures, the same technique is used on the anterior and lateral abdominal sides to strengthen the fascias concerned. The return to the starting position is passive to avoid concentric action. The protocol implements the rules to determine its effectiveness: very slowly and with low intensity in the initial stages, these two parameters being gradually intensified strictly according to absence of pain during and between sessions: the ROM very gradually integrating into the sector of maximum elongation [50, 71].

3.7.2.2 The Second Phase

The second phase involves strengthening the abdominal muscles (cladding) and the spinal and hip extensors the deficits of which are frequently associated.

Eccentric adductor work continues with intensification. Indeed, the eccentric muscle loads have been the basis of our treatment of tendon injuries since the work of Stanish et al. [51]. The tendon structure must also receive appropriate training to improve its mechanical and protect against microlesions resulting from external constraints.

The exercise incorporates the resilient elongation parameters of the musculotendinous unit (according to a defined ROM), speed of movement, and intensity of contraction. The selected joint displacement integrates with the maximum elongation sector (external course) as soon as possible.

To achieve this eccentric work, use of an isokinetic dynamometer has many advantages, as it enables quantified control of the resistance and speed, optimal contraction due to the auto-adaptive resistance, instant feedback, individualization of the workload, and control of the ROM.

The effectiveness of eccentric work in the treatment of tendon injuries has been regularly demonstrated over the last few decades [49, 50, 52] (Barthélémy et al. 2014).

If isokinetic equipment is the modality of choice for technique building, the eccentric rehabilitative exercises can be delivered through the use of different devices: manual application by the physiotherapist, use of direct charges or mobilized by ropes or chains, elastic resistance. Each category presents advantages and limitations regarding the availability and the cost of equipment, the efficiency and specificity of training, and patient safety. However, the management of the adductor longus tendinopathy need the implementation of this eccentric work protocol.

3.7.2.3 The Third Phase

The third phase includes the neuromuscular reprogramming form of muscle activation with pelvic stabilization exercises for the abdominal and lower limbs, first on balancing trays.

The objective of this phase is to develop a good lower abdominal muscle synergy between the pelvis and limbs and to improve muscle control and balance. During this phase we can use a work on the Klein ball, and the Pau-Toronto protocol [53]. Sports with many alternate unipedal movements benefit greatly from this phase. This stage continues on the ground, where the work will be more specific to the sport practiced: the movement is first to be made in the center and if no pain or when the 80 % threshold in a painless maximum eccentric contraction is reached they will become a real preparation for the sporting gesture. The development of aerobic capacity and the maximal aerobic power and finally the support work (changes in direction, front-back race, shuffle) are part of the last part of this phase.

3.7.2.4 The Fourth Phase

The fourth and final phase is the continuation of specific movements for recovery, still without pain. This is a true program of progressive reintegration into the team. Monthly medical monitoring is necessary to address adductor longus fissural rebel tendinopathy. Platelet-rich plasma infiltration (PRP) could represent a therapeutic hope following the results of various in vitro and animal experiments [74]. The addition of eccentric loads in the aftermath of the injection of PRP improves the efficiency of this type of treatment [54].

3.7.3 Surgical Treatment

The surgical treatment consists of a tenotomy under general anesthesia. An incision of about 3 cm is made. After dissection of the superficial plans, the adductor longus tendon component is resected and pushed down (sometimes using pliers if an old calcific tendinopathy) until there is a soft area measuring 3–4 cm. The femoral fascia and the subcutaneous tissue are closed. The postoperative course is simple, with few bruising complications (2 %) and little infection (0.05 %) [72].

Adhesions occur in 15–25 % of cases, usually within a month or 3 months of surgery. After an adductor longus tenotomy, mobilization of the hip from the first attempt to lift by the patient is required, to prevent adhesions between the tendon and femoral fascia, which burden this surgery [55]. The patient needs to practice hip movements such as active abduction, flexion, extension, and rotation, avoiding active contraction of the adductors, which is painful at this stage.

The practice of administering manual eccentric loads to the adductor gradually facilitates the healing of tendons by collagen stimulation and prevents scar adhesions.

Rehabilitation takes place in several stages. Walking is allowed from the day after surgery if no or light pain. Static exercises can be considered as soon as possible within the first week. During the second and third weeks, a straight course is recommended: running very slow stopping when there is pain, with 1 or 2 days of rest between sessions. In parallel to this work, abdominal strengthening is gradually increased. During the fourth week, rehabilitation of the abdominal wall and groin is intensified with the implementation of a program of re-athletization.

The specific training for a return to sport is progressive and controlled, postponing ball-striking until around the 45th day.

A combination of ductal forms and chronic lesions of the adductor insertion is common [56]: 55 out of 80 soccer players according to Rifi et al. in 2009 [57]. In the experience of Reboul, in a retrospective series of 180 patients operated on for tendinopathy adductor, 80 % of patients had associated parietal failure requiring surgical treatment [31].

Surgical treatment is very effective for abdominal pathologies, which are often resistant to medical treatment. In the case of an abdominal pure form or a proven mixed form, surgery becomes necessary if rest and rehabilitation care for the duration of 2 months do not allow sports recovery [58].

The two most frequently used surgical techniques in athletes are [14]:

- Nesovic, the principle of which is a bilateral tensioning of the broad muscles of the abdomen by lowering of the inguinal ligament.
- Shouldice, administered to fight against the enlargement of the inguinal canal using a suture in three planes: the transverse fascia is retightened using an overcoat suture between the inguinal ligament and the conjoint tendon, closing the aponeurosis of the abdominal external oblique muscle.

The results obtained were good or very good in 80–90 % of cases.

A minimal repair technique exists: using endoscopy only, opening the transverse fascia and doubling the reverse fascia. The indication is only for a light deficiency of the abdominal posterior wall, with no pain of longus adductor insertion.

In our opinion, endoscopic single-shutter techniques with prosthetic reinforcements, which are practiced by visceral surgeons, do not have a place in athletes, because they do not meet the aim of rebalancing the constraints of the pubic symphysis.

3.8 Prevention

Adductor tendinopathy is very common in an athlete's life. It is the result of intrinsic factors such as postural dysfunction, hyperlordosis, a weakness of the abdominals. Extrinsic factors can also set off the tendinopathy. Indeed, overtraining is a strong element leading to stress. Furthermore, soft fields may be a factor.

Primary prevention is identifying subjects at risk: deficiency in the abdominal wall with dehiscence or Malgaigne's sign: oblique protrusion, ROM limitation of the hip, anteversion of the pelvis [59]. An improvement program with regard to these weak points will have to be made throughout the individual's career to avoid possible decompensation. Prevention of this consists of four forms of groin pain, not to mention the prevention of extrinsic factors including: the effective management of workloads, suitable muscle building, and avoiding abdominal work that involves significant increases in intra-abdominal pressure.

The frequency of groin pain has declined sharply among top athletes over the past 15 years, whereas it has increased in other disciplines and among amateur athletes [60]. This is undoubtedly because of prevention programs that are now in place and systematically applied at the highest level. However, they must be reviewed regularly, as with any prevention program, by medical staff, technicians, and by athletes themselves, so that they do not reoffend. This is especially true as training and competition increase in frequency and intensity.

According to some studies, a significant recurrence rate has been reported in professional team sports: 38 and 44% [11, 12], and 25–32% of professional players suffer a recurrence during the season [61]. The prevention programs should take into account the training load, the morphotype, potential imbalances between the stabilizing muscles of the pelvis and hip, loss of ROM or abnormalities of the hip joint.

It is important to understand the function of the adductor complex; they mainly aid hip adduction and the thigh rotations (lateral or medial, according to the muscles and parts). Thus, it is essential to consider the rotator aspect of this muscular complex. We find this injury more frequently in collective sports such as soccer, basketball, handball, all requiring explosivity, acceleration, deceleration, and rotation. In soccer, the adductors participate in passing and shooting too. Here is a way of preventing adductor tendinopathy.

First of all, during the pre-season, some evaluations can be made to determine a player's profile. Postural tests and screening are fundamental [62]. The static posture is observed, then the dynamic posture through assessment using the National Academy of Sports Medicine's overhead squat test and the single-leg squat test. These tests enable us to determine any imbalances and compensations. Each dysfunction is linked to underactive muscles and overactive muscles. The Functional Movement Screen [63] can be used too. These kinds of tests provide information that can explain recurrent injuries or risks of injuries (i.e., the knee valgus and the risk of an ACL tear). Here are few examples of dysfunctions and imbalances that increase the risks of developing an adductor tendinopathy: hyperlordosis with weak core muscles (especially the external oblique muscle), a weak gluteus maximus, and a weak gluteus medius.

Second, there is the lower-crossed syndrome, showing the link with the weak gluteus, weak abdominals and tight hip flexors, and a tight erector spinae (causing the hyperlordosis). The relationship between the weakness of abdominals and the adductor tendinopathy is well known. During activity, the core plays important role in balancing the body, maintaining the pelvis (and forcing transmission, resisting contact…). If the core is weak, the body compensates by over-activating the peripheral muscles as adductors or hamstrings, and could lead to tendinopathy.

Third, mobility is a key in the prevention of any injury (especially in the groin area). We know that soccer players have a limited ROM of the hips owing to the particular role of the adductors [64]. Many mobility exercises and stretching postures exist to fight stiffness and to reduce the risk of developing inflammation.

Fourth, proprioception should be included in the protocol of prevention for adductors. Indeed, the adductors are tonic, i.e., they contribute to maintaining the posture. They should be worked in any situation (including rotations) to reduce the risk of inflammation.

Strengthening is essential for prevention. There are two ways to prevent the adductor tendinopathy. The first one is by strengthening the adductor complex (brevis, magnus, longus, pectineus, and gracilis) and the hips flexor complex, both in eccentric mode [51, 65–68]. The manual work can be undertaken by physiotherapists. Bodyweight and machines also help to strengthen these muscles. We repeat that the eccentric mode, which is used mainly for lengthening and stretching, should be reserved for these muscles. It should be added that training with an elastic band is not very interesting for the adductor complex because the resistance with bands exists mainly in the internal course (when the insertions get closer), whereas we look for the lengthening of the muscles. The second goal is global strengthening. The main idea here is to increase the strength of the gluteus and of the core to stabilize the pelvis and the trunk to release the over-tension of the adductor complex.

Last, the management of the training load is very useful for preventing all kinds of stress injuries, such as tendinopathies. Medical and technical staff must work together to define the limits and risks for each player. Many methods exist to control the training load through subjective tests (questions, rating of perceived exertion [RPE], feelings, sleep, fatigue, etc.), and/or objective tests such as heart rate variability [69, 70].

Here are some examples for preventing adductor tendinopathy:

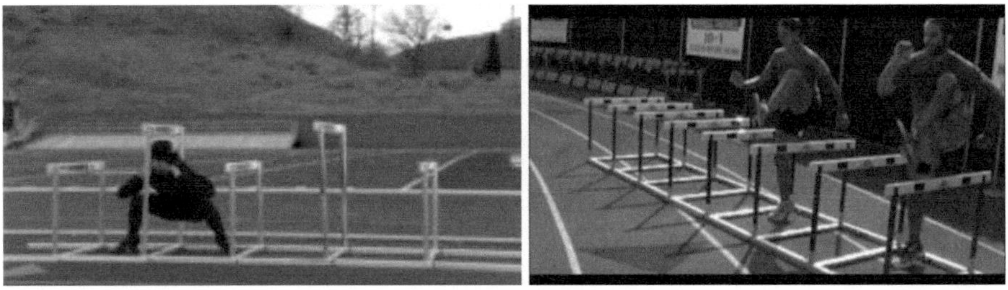

Hip mobility

- Mobility: static deep squats, hurdle crossing:
  - Stretching, and myofascial release with a foam roller. For adductors, hip flexors, erector spinae (if hyperlordosis)
  - Eccentric strengthening of the adductors: lying with bent knees, lying with straight legs, seated; with manual resistance, with bodyweight through lateral lunges (using a slider pad), with machines
  - Eccentric strengthening of the hip flexors: with manual resistance, or bodyweight, or an additional load
  - Global strengthening of the adductors: sumo squat, sumo deadlift, split squat, lunges, step-ups
  - Strengthening of the gluteus maximus: with hip extension, hip thrusts, or through global movements such as deep squats or as a deadlift. Strengthening of the gluteus medius: lying on the side and hip abduction, lateral movements with an elastic band over the knees as lateral steps, or as lateral lunges, or even global movements described above, with an elastic band
- Core training: front and lateral planks and all variations (static or dynamic; with med-ball or physio-ball). Specific work on the oblique muscle can be added.
- Proprioception: single-leg stance with many situations, surfaces, static or dynamic, closed or open-eyed, manipulation of tools, rotations, etc.

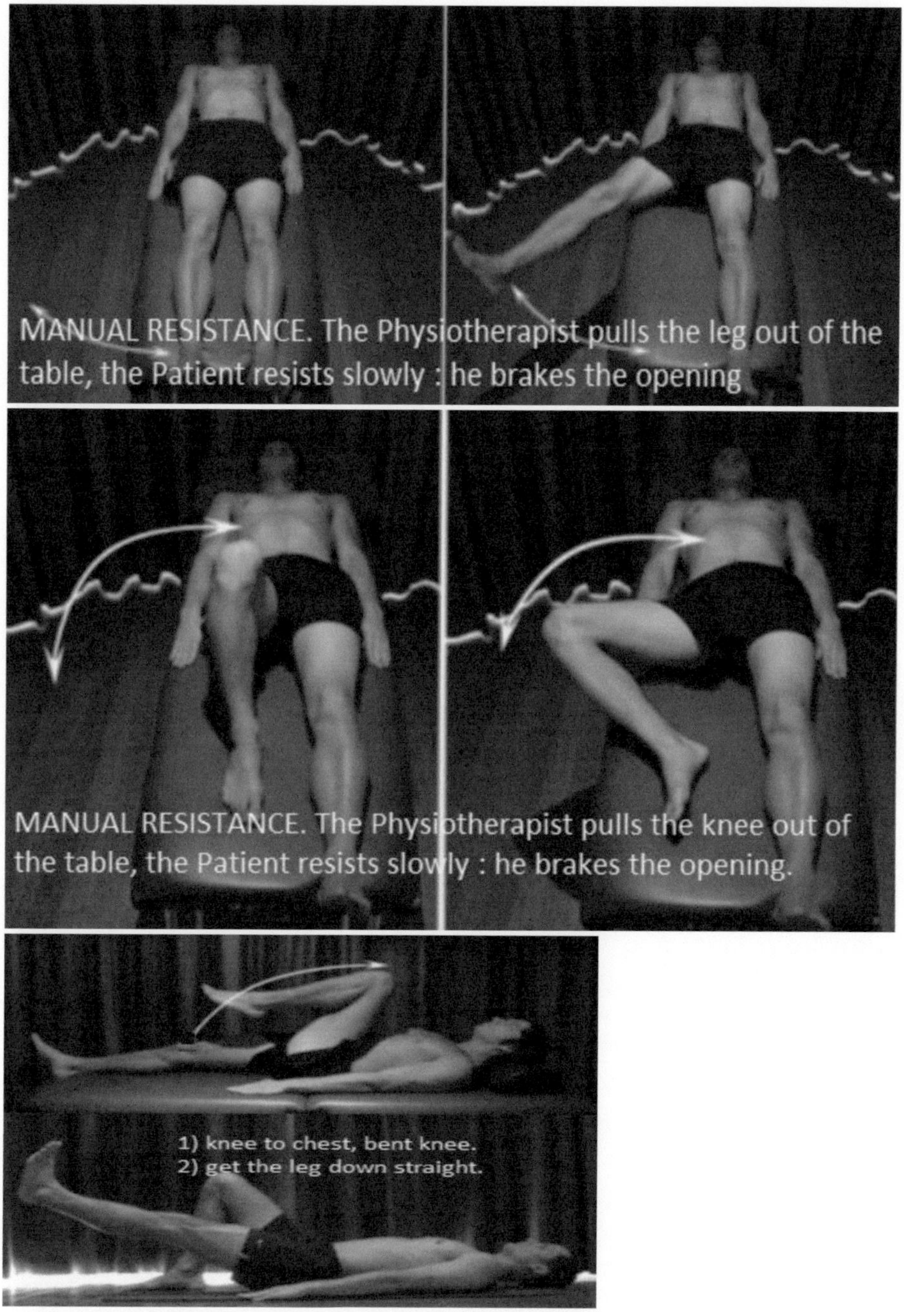

Let us have a look now at an example of rehabilitation for this kind of injury. We talk about conditioning and the ball parts. We add treatment and strengthening before and/ or after these sessions with exercises as explained previously. Here is a proposed a session: players warm up on a bicycle, then perform a specific protocol for the adductor complex (manual exercises with physiotherapists, or on a isokinetic dynamometer, or a machine). After that, they warm up on a field with skills, before starting the field program that follows. The last part of the session is in the gym with global strengthening, a core work-out, stretching or self-myofascial release. After a number of sessions of eccentric work, the players are able to start running. Players first run for progressively longer periods: 10 min, 2 × 10 min, 2 × 15 min. Then, we introduce accelerations; progressively, day after day, the players have to accelerate within the width of the box, then within the width of the field, and then within the length of the field. We introduce the ball during that period, with easy technical workouts first. Day after day, players perform circuits with more or less intensity. The next step is the intensity: players carry out interval training (2 × 8 min, 10 s at maximal aerobic velocity/20 s passive recovery). In the same period, the ball workouts gain in importance, and are more intensive for conditioning and muscles. In the field program, we mean running and ball workouts, and the players have to realize in all situations that they live in a game: running at different speeds, with changes in direction, rotations, accelerations/decelerations, driving the ball, passes, contacts, jumps, etc. At any time during the protocol, we control the training load and adjust the sessions if necessary.

3.9 Synthesis and Therapeutic Indications

Inguinal pain is very common in sport, but among many diagnoses, adductor insertion tendinopathy is one of the four most common entities either in the associated or isolated form. Our purpose was to detail clinical, etiological, and therapeutic plans, while providing the criteria by which to eliminate other pathological conditions. Under

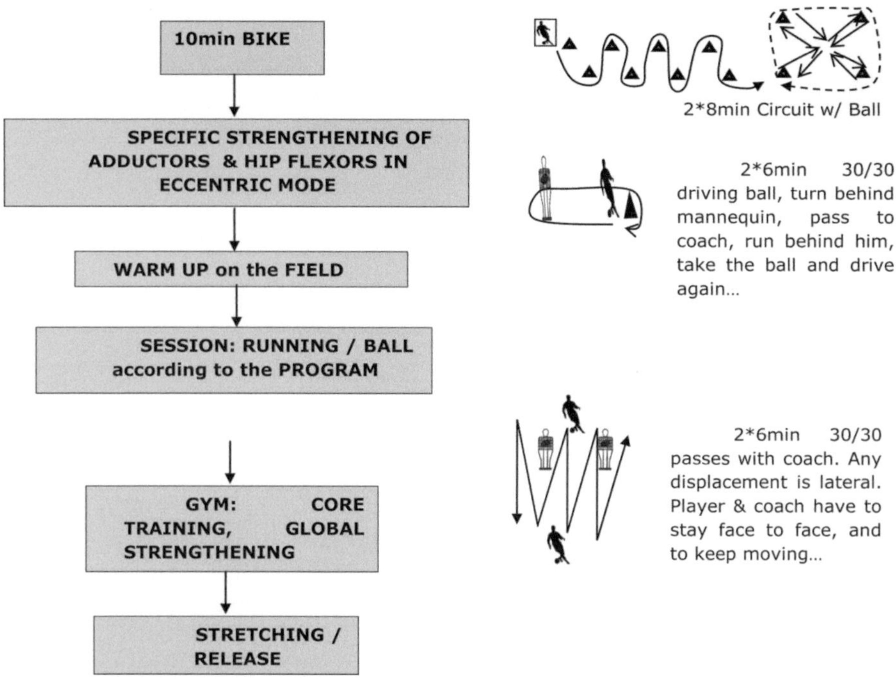

these conditions it is essential to establish as soon as possible a specific positive diagnosis. Early consultation is crucial; it is easy in professional clubs with a medical staff present, but it is more difficult for amateur athletes who may be extremely hampered in their physical activities or in everyday life to consult a physician.

3.9.1 Subject Seen Early: Acute Mode

- Confirm the diagnosis of adductor longus enthesopathy by pain at palpation, adductor stretching, and painful adduction resistance
- No pain at the hip flexors and trunk to eliminate rectus abdominis tendinopathy or athletic pubalgia with in this case a pain when coughing after effort and a painful inguinal ring that expands on impulsive coughing
- No limitation of hip amplitudes for eliminating arthropathy
- No pain on FADIR to eliminate FAI

Treatment consists of rest, bicycle riding, manual eccentric movements in the internal course without pain during and after increasing the intensity, ROM, and speed gradually one single criterion at a time. When the external position is reached, painless recovery on the ground is possible.

3.9.2 Subject Seen Late: Chronic Mode

Confirmation of the diagnosis is much more difficult because of the spread of pain due to the chronicity and anatomical intricacy of the neighboring structures. At first, the pathological hip condition should be eliminated.

Clinically, pain includes:

- Palpation of the adductor longus insertion
- Lodge adductor roughly contracted
- Limited and painful lodge stretching (FABER)
- Resisting adduction
- Resisting hip flexion
- Resisted trunk flexion
- Palpation of the rectus abdominis insertion on the pubis
- Testing of the contralateral adductor

but the absence of impulsivity to affirm the isolated form. Although this is rare at this stage, the frequency of the association between chronic enthesopathy of the adductor and the weakness of the posterior wall is very high [31].

Treatment is associated with NSAIDs, stretching, and eccentric loads of slow speed limiting the ROM in a nonpainful area, low intensity, gradually increasing the criteria and respecting the rule of indolence, using the same protocol on hip flexors and trunk and rotators, manually then with an isokinetic dynamometer to follow a numerical progression of evolution and allow the resumption of running with objective criteria. Ultrasound and MRI clarify the degree of tendon damage and eliminate or not the associated forms. Two injections of PRP at 3-week intervals associated with eccentric submaximal work may allow complete pain relief in less than 2 months. After resuming racing, the increase in physical activity is highly codified. The collaboration among physician, physiotherapist, and medical trainer is essential for the full recovery of the player.

In the case of failure: persistent pain after 2 months despite well performed treatment and in the case of a deficit of wall association, surgery is programmed with only a superficial tenotomy [14, 58, 73] or associated with abdominal wall strengthening using the Shouldice technique.

3.10 Conclusion

Groin tendinopathy is a difficult disease requiring good clinical knowledge. It is part of one of the four groin syndromes of sportsmen: adductor enthesopathy, rectus abdominis enthesopathy, posterior abdominal wall weakness, and pubic osteoarthropathy. It may be isolated, but is often associated with other clinical forms. The diagnosis should specify the various forms of damage so that treatment is appropriate: conservative and medical in isolated forms, often surgical in associated forms after the failure of medical treatment within 2–3 months, especially when treatment was delayed. The identification of subjects at risk is crucial in professional sports, but impractical in amateur sports. Information in sporting circles and in the general public on the importance of early medical consultation in this type of pathological condition would be a very good thing.

References

1. Maffulli N, Renstrom P, Leadbetter WB (2005) Part 1 Tendon injuries, vol 5, Basic science and clinical medicine. Springer, London, pp 32–35
2. Werner J, Hägglund M, Waldén M, Ekstrand J (2009) UEFA injury study: a prospective study of hip and groin injuries in professional football over seven consecutive seasons. Br J Sports Med 43(13):1036–1040
3. Gilmore J (1998) Groin pain in the soccer athlete: fact, fiction, and treatment. Clin Sports Med 17(4):787–793
4. Ekstrand J, Hilding J (1999) The incidence and differential diagnosis of acute groin injuries in male soccer players. Scand J Med Sci Sports 9(2):98–103
5. Kaux JF, Forthomme B, Goff CL, Crielaard JM, Croisier JL (2011) Current opinions on tendinopathy. J Sports Med Sci 10(2):238
6. Valent A, Frizziero A, Bressan S, Zanella E, Giannotti E, Masiero S (2012) Insertional tendinopathy of the adductors and rectus abdominis in athletes: a review. Muscles Ligaments Tendons J 2:142–148

7. Robertson BA, Barker PJ, Fahrer M, Schache AG (2009) The anatomy of the pubic region revisited: implications for the pathogenesis and clinical management of chronic groin pain in athletes. Sports Med 39(3):225–234
8. Tuite DJ, Finegan PJ, Saliaris AP, Renstrom PA, Donne B, O'Brien M (1998) Anatomy of the proximal musculotendinous junction of the adductor longus muscle. Knee Surg Sports Traumatol Arthrosc 6:134–137
9. Strauss EJ, Campbell K, Bosco JA (2007) Analysis of the cross-sectional area of the adductor longus tendon: a descriptive anatomic study. Am J Sports Med 35:996–999
10. Zoga AC, Kavanagh EC, Omar IM et al (2008) Athletic pubalgia and the "sports hernia": MR imaging findings. Radiology 247(3):797–807
11. McIntyre J, Johnson C, Schroeder EL (2006) Groin pain in athletes. Curr Sports Med Rep 5:293–299
12. Tyler TF, Silvers HJ, Gerhardt MB et al (2010) Groin injuries in sports medicine. Sport Health 20:1–6
13. Bisciotti GN, Auci A, Di Marzo F, Galli R, Pulici L, Carimati G, Quaglia A, Volpi P (2015) Groin pain syndrome: an association of different pathologies and a case of presentation. Muscles Ligaments Tendons J 5(3):214–222
14. Bouvard M, Lippa A, Reboul G (2011) Pubalgie du sportif. Appareil locomoteur, 14-323-A-10. Elsevier Masson SAS, Paris
15. Sailly M (2013) La pubalgie du sportif en pratique. Sci Sport 28(4):225–232
16. Thorborg K, Holmich P (2013) Advancing hip and groin injury management: from eminence to evidence. Br J Sports Med 43:602–605
17. Orchard JW, Read JW, Neophyton J (1998) Groin pain associated with ultrasound findings of inguinal canal posterior wall deficiency in Australian rules footballers. Br J Sports Med 23:141–145
18. Ferret JM (2012) La hanche du sportif: l'œil du terrain in Sport et vieillissement articulaire avec arthrose précoce et conflit antérieur de hanche. Revue de chirurgie orthopédique et traumatologique 98:313–314
19. Bouvard M, Lippa A, Reboul G, Lutz C (2012) Mise au point: La pubalgie du sportif. J Traumatol Sport 29:105–128
20. Weir A, de Vos RJ, Moen M, Hölmich P, Tol JL (2011) Prevalence of radiological signs of femoroacetabular impingement in patients presenting with long-standing adductor-related groin pain. Br J Sports Med 45:6–9
21. Nepple JJ, Brophy RH, Matava MJ, Wright RW, Clohisy JC (2012) Radiographic findings of femoroacetabular impingement in National Football League combine athletes undergoing radiographs for previous hip or groin pain. Arthroscopy 28:1396–1403
22. Allen D, Beaulé PE, Ramadan O, Doucette S (2009) Prevalence of associated deformities and hip pain in patients with cam-type femoroacetabular impingement. J Bone Joint Surg Br 91:589–594
23. Bonin N, Tanji PH (2012) Sport et conflit: relation entre conflit et lésions articulaires.in Sport et vieillissement articulaire avec arthrose précoce et conflit antérieur de hanche. Revue de chirurgie orthopédique et traumatologique 98:315–317
24. Agricola R, Bessems JH, Ginai AZ, Heijboer MP et al (2012) The development of Cam-type deformity in the adolescent and young male soccer players. Am J Sports Med 40(5): 1099–1106
25. Ganz R, Parvizi J, Beck M, Leunig M, Nötzli H, Siebenrock KA (2003) Femoroacetabular impingement: a cause for osteoarthritis of the hip. Clin Orthop Relat Res 417:112–120
26. Siebenrock K, Ferner F, Noble P, Santore R, Werlen S, Mamisch TC (2011) The cam-type deformity of the proximal femur arises in childhood in response to vigorous sporting activity. Clin Orthop Relat Res 469:3229–3240
27. Murray RO, Duncan C (1971) Athletic activity in adolescence as an etiological factor in degenerative hip disease. J Bone Joint Surg Br 53(3):406–419

28. Philippon MJ, Weiss DR, Kuppersmith DA, Briggs KK, Hay CJ (2010) Arthroscopic labral repair and treatment of femoroacetabular impingement in professional hockey players. Am J Sports Med 38:99–104
29. Siebenrock KA, Schoeniger R, Ganz R (2003) Anterior femoro-acetabular impingement due to acetabular retroversion. Treatment with periacetabular osteotomy. J Bone Joint Surg Am 85:278–286
30. Morales-Conde S, Socas M, Barranco A (2010) Sportsmen hernia: what do we know? Hernia 14:515
31. Pesquer L, Reboul G, Dallaudiere B, Meyer P (2013) Imagerie de la tendinopâthie des adducteurs. In: Actualités en échographie de l'appareil locomoteur. Sauramps Medical Ed, Montpellier, pp 55–64
32. Riley G (2004) The pathogenesis of tendinopathy. A molecular perspective. Rheumatology 43:131–142
33. Estwanik JJ, Sloane B, Rosemberg MA (1988) Groin strain and other possible causes of groin pain. Phys Sport Med 19:59–65
34. Puig PL, Trove P, Savalli L (2004) La pubalgie: du diagnostic au retour sur le terrain. Ann Readpt Med Phys 47(6):356–364
35. Orchard J, Read JW, Verrall GM, Slavotinek JP (2000) Pathophysiology of chronic pain in the athlete. ISMJ 1(1)
36. Nicolas SJ, Tyler TF (2002) Adductor muscle strains in sport. Sports Med 5:339–344
37. Busquet L (2013) Traitement préventif pour diminuer la fréquence des pubalgies: analyse de la méthode des chaînes physiologiques. Kiné Actualité 1341:18–23
38. Seiller M, Mathieu R, Ferret JM (1990) Morphotype du footballeur: constat clinique à partir d'une population de joueurs professionnels. Sports Med 44:1–8
39. Ferret JM (2007) Prévention de la pubalgie. Compte rendu Congrès Pubalgie Bordeaux
40. Holmich P, Holmich LR, Bjerg AM (2004) Clinical examination of athletes with groin pain: an intraobserver and interobserver reliability study. Br J Sports Med 38:446–451
41. Weir A, Jansen J, van Keulen J, Mens J, Backx F, Stam H (2010) Short and mid-term results of a comprehensive treatment program for longstanding adductor-related groin pain in athletes: a case series. Phys Ther Sport 11(3):99–103
42. Lowell G, Galloway H, Hopkins W, Harvey A (2006) Osteitis pubis and assessment of bone marrow edema at the pelvic symphysis with MRI in a elite junior man soccer quad. Clin J Sports Med 16:117–122
43. Brennan D, O'Connell MJ, Ryan M, Cunningham P, Taylor D, Cronin C et al (2005) Secondary cleft sign as a marker of injury in athletes with groin pain: MR image appearance and interpretation. Radiology 235:162–167
44. Pesquer L, Reboul G, Silvestre A, Poussange N, Meyer P, Dallaudiere B (2015) Imaging of adductor-related groin pain. Diagn Interv Imaging 96(9):861–869
45. Brasseur JL, Laulom JP (2013) Pubalgie: apport de l'échographie. J Traumatol Sport 30:36–41
46. Peetrons P (2007) les pubalgies: approche par l'échographie. In: Bassin et Hanche. Monographies de la SIMS. Sauramps Medical Ed, Montpellier, pp 179–183
47. Jansen JA, Mens JM, Backx FJ et al (2008) Treatment of longstanding groin pain in athletes: a systematic review. Scand J Med Sci Sports 18:263–274
48. Holmich P, Uhrskou P, Ulnits L et al (1999) Effectiveness of active physical training as a treatment for longstanding adductor –related groin pain in athletes: randomized trial. Lancet 353:439–443
49. Fyfe I, Stanish WD (1992) The use of eccentric training and stretching in the treatment and prevention of tendon injuries. Clin Sports Med 11(3):601–624
50. Queiros Da Silva C, Cotte T, Vicard L, Chantelot L, Ferret JM (2005) Interest of eccentric isokinetic exercises in cases of calcaneal tendinosis and thigh muscular injuries prospective study results. Isok Exerc Sci 13:39–44
51. Stanish WD, Rubinovich RM, Curwin S (1986) Eccentric exercise in chronic tendinitis. Clin Orthop Relat Res 208:65–68

52. Jensen J, Hölmich P, Bandholm T, Zebis MK, Andersen LL, Thorborg K (2014) Eccentric strengthening effect of hip adductor training with elastic bands in soccer players: a randomized controlled trial. Br J Sports Med 48(4):332–338
53. Bouvard M, Dorochenko P, Lanusse P, Duraffour H (2004) La Pubalgie du sportif: stratégie thérapeutique. Revue de la littérature et proposition d'un protocole de rééducation. J Traumatol Sport 21:146–163
54. Kaux JF, Crielaard JM (2013) Platelet-rich-plasma application in the management of chronic tendinopathies. Acta Orthop Belg 79:10–15
55. Le Picard P, Reboul G, Vuckovic Z (2013) Mise au point: le traitement chirurgical des pubalgies. Sci Sport 28:233–238
56. Le Gall F (1993) la pubalgie du sportif. A propos de 214 cas. Thèse de médecine Rennes
57. Rifi M, Muller J, Mezghani S, Londero A, Jaeger JH (2009) Intervention de Nesovic dans le traitement des pubalgies chez le footballeur. A propos d'une série de 80 cas. J Traumatol Sport 26:81–84
58. Thomas JG, Kaitlin M, Carroll BS, Amun M, Andrew JW, Guillaume BS, Dumont D, Randy MC (2014) Surgical technique for treatment of recalcitrant adductor longus tendinopathy. Arthrosc Tech 3(2):e293–e297
59. Orchard JW (2015) Men at higher risk of groin injuries in elite team sports: a systematic review. Br J Sports Med 49(12):798–802
60. Rochcongar P (2013) Prévention de la pubalgie. In: Acquisition en médecine physique et de Réadaptation. Prévention des troubles musculo-squelettiques chez le sportif. Sauramps Medical Ed, Montpellier, pp 130–134
61. Gibbon WW (1999) Groin pain in athletes. Lancet 353(9162):1444–1445
62. McCall A (2015) Injury risk factors, screening tests and preventive strategies: a systematic review on the evidence that underpins the perception and practices of 44 soccer teams from various premier leagues. Br J Sports Med 49:583–589
63. Gray Cook (2014) Functional Movement Screening: the use of fundamental movements as an assessment of function, Part 1. The International Journal of Sports Physical Therapy. 9(3):396.
64. Ibrahim A, Murrell GA, Knapman P (2007) Adductor strain and hip range of movement in male professional soccer players. J Orthopaedic Surg 15(1):46–49
65. Stanish WD (1984) Overuse injuries in athletes: a perspective. Med Sci Sports Exerc 16(1):1–7
66. Middleton P, Montero C (2004) Eccentric muscular contraction: implications in treatment of athletes. Ann Readapt Med Phys 47(6):282–289
67. Frizziero A et al (2014) The role of eccentric in sport injuries rehabilitation. Br Med Bull 110:47–75
68. Rees JD et al (2009) Eccentric exercises; why do they work, what are the problems and how can we improve them. Br J Sports Med 43:242–246
69. Aubert AE (2003) Heart rate variability in athletes. Sports Med 33(12):889–919
70. Baumert M (2006) Heart rate variability, blood pressure variability, and baroreflex sensitivity in overtrained athletes. Clin J Sport Med 16(5):412–417
71. Barthelemy Y, Kaux JF, Ferret JM (2014). Isocinétisme et sport de haut niveau: Applications à la traumatologie du sport. Scinece et Motricité 85:77–91.
72. Gill TJ, Carroll KM, Makani A, Wall AJ, Dumont GD, Cohn RM (2014) Surgical technique for treatment of recalcitrant adductor longus tendinopathy. Arthrosc Techn 3(2):e293–e297
73. Reboul G (2014) La chirurgie de la tendinopathie des adducteurs. Congrès 1ère journée européenne de la Pubalgie. Clinique du Sport Bordeaux Merignac. Bordeaux
74. Dallaudière B, Lempicki M, Pesquer L, Louedec L, Preux PM, Meyer P, Hummel V, Larbi A, Deschamps L, Journe C, Hess A. Silvestre A, Sargos P, Loriaut P, Boyer P (2013). Efficacité de l'injection intra-tendineuse du plasma riche en plaquettes dans le traitement tendinosis: évaluation globale d'un modèle de rat. Eur Radiol 23:2830.

Chapter 4
Rectus Femoris Tendinopathy

Stefano Dragoni and Andrea Bernetti

Abstract Rectus femoris tendinopathies are not particularly frequent occurrences in sports traumatology.

It is possible to observe their presence in sports activities requiring strong, repeated, and eccentric loading with maximal lengthening in lower limbs such as during sprinting and kicking.

The symptoms show a gradual and progressive onset of pain and discomfort in the anterior aspect of the hip and are typically aggravated by exercise especially during jumping and running.

Patient history and clinical evaluation, including direct palpation of the tendon and resisted muscle activation, are essential to make the appropriate diagnosis.

Imaging is helpful in confirming diagnosis. Ultrasound and magnetic resonance provide valuable diagnostic information, useful for planning therapeutic strategies.

Conservative treatment includes oral and topical anti-inflammatory drugs and physical therapy with a wide variety of modalities available.

Surgical treatment is unnecessary in most cases; surgery may be a valuable option in selected patients who have failed 3–6 months of conservative treatment or in painful calcific tendinopathy.

4.1 Introduction

Overuse disorders of tendons, bones, and joints represent a widespread problem in sport and a challenge to sports physicians. Achilles, patellar, and supraspinatus tendons are often site of overuse injuries, while rectus femoris (RF) tendinopathies are not so often observed in the clinical practice of sport medicine [1].

S. Dragoni, MD (✉) • A. Bernetti, MD
Institute of Sport Medicine and Science, Italian Olympic Committee, Rome, Italy
e-mail: stefano.dragoni@coni.it

G.N. Bisciotti, P. Volpi (eds.), *The Lower Limb Tendinopathies*,
Sports and Traumatology, DOI 10.1007/978-3-319-33234-5_4

Tendinopathy is an umbrella term that indicates that there is a non-rupture injury in the tendon or paratendon, which is exacerbated by mechanical loading and may lead to long-lasting disability [2].

In athletes, rectus femoris muscle/tendon acute injuries have a high incidence; indeed they are second only to the hamstrings tear among lower extremity acute injuries.

Rectus femoris acute injuries are common in soccer players because the athletic kicking motion involves forceful eccentric contraction while passively stretched at the onset of the forward swing phase.

The strong eccentric loading with maximal lengthening during sprinting and kicking predisposes the rectus femoris to injury. Although proximal injuries are mainly myotendinous or myoaponeurotic, proximal tendon avulsions or ruptures may also be seen, involving direct, indirect, or both tendons. Indirect tendon complete or partial tears have been reported to be more frequent than direct and conjoined tendon injuries. It has been proposed that proximal rectus femoris insertional injuries may progress from the indirect to the direct head and then to the conjoined tendon [3, 4].

The same mechanism of acute injury in a skeletally immature athlete could result in an avulsion fracture of the anterior inferior iliac spine (AIIS) at the origin of the direct head, owing to the vulnerability of the open apophysis, while the same gesture in adults, performed with high intensity for repeated time, may lead to tendinopathy [5].

4.2 Anatomy and Functional Anatomy

The rectus femoris is the most superficial and the only biarticular muscle of the quadriceps group. Its proximal insertion is complex, with two main proximal origins.

The direct or straight tendon is located at the anterior hip, arising from the anterior inferior iliac spine (AIIS) and forming the anterior aponeurosis.

The indirect or reflected tendon is located at the anterolateral hip, arising from the superior acetabular ridge and posterior coxofemoral capsule, and forms the deep central aponeurosis, extending up to the lower third of the muscle. The two heads unite at an acute angle and form the conjoined tendon around 2 cm distal to their origin (Fig. 4.1). A third and inconsistent head may arise from the inferior edge of the indirect tendon, attached superficially to the gluteus minimus muscle and deeply to the lateral iliofemoral ligament [6–8].

Sometimes, between the straight tendon and AIIS, there can be, although not constantly, the interposition of a bursa.

The tendon, devoid of synovial sheath and covered by peritendon, presents morphological and structural characteristics comparable to those of similar anatomical structures as the Achilles or quadriceps tendon.

Usually the integration of tendon into the bone occurs at a specialized interface known as *enthesis*, through a multitissue interface [9].

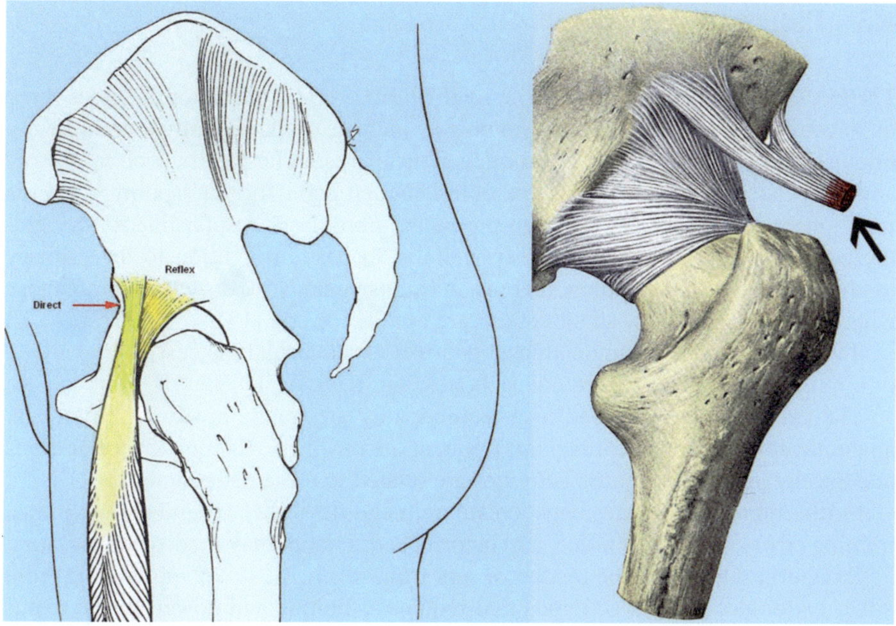

Fig. 4.1 On the left, direct and reflex tendon of rectus femoris; on the right, conjoined tendon (*black arrow*)

Tendons and ligaments may attach to the bone via either fibrous or fibrocartilaginous insertions which are more common than fibrous.

The straight tendon of rectus femoris muscle belongs in its junctional site to the fibrocartilaginous entheses with four transitional layers from the bone to tendon; the first zone, distal to bone-tendon junction, consists of tendon and is populated by fibroblasts; the second zone consists of uncalcified fibrocartilage which is populated by fibrochondrocytes; the third is composed of mineralized fibrocartilage; and the fourth consists of bone [10].

Concerning functional aspects, electrophysiological studies have shown that the rectus femoris muscle functions independently from the vastus muscles during walking. It extends the knee, flexes strongly the hip, and stabilizes the pelvis on the femur during weightbearing. These anatomical specificities, together with the strong eccentric loading with maximal lengthening during sprinting and kicking, may predispose the rectus femoris to acute and overuse injuries as mentioned before [3, 11, 12].

4.3 Pathophysiology

The classic description of the tensile load-bearing region of tendon includes three main components: (1) type I collagen fibers which are predominantly longitudinally oriented, (2) a well-hydrated, non-collagenous extracellular matrix (rich in glycosaminoglycans), (3) and cells. The predominant cell population in healthy tendon is traditionally categorized as collagen-producing fibroblasts, responsible for the synthesis of the collagen fibers and extracellular matrix. In addition to the primary load-bearing part of the tendon, there is an extensive network of septae (endotenon) where the nerves and few small vessels are mainly located [13].

The main cause of tendinopathies is overuse, as the result of excessive, repetitive, or improper overloads to the tendons, bones, and joints.

The causes that could lead to a tendinopathy are many, involving biological, anatomical, and mechanical factors; frequent actions involving quick accelerations and decelerations or eccentric activities are related to these pathologies [14].

Furthermore, imbalances between strength and flexibility around certain joints, training errors, faulty technique, and incorrect equipment may predispose to injury.

Structural damage to the tendon occurs from repetitive strain and loading from either endurance or skill activities that require technique and power. In the rectus femoris tendon, overuse acts usually through kicking and explosive movements as in sprint starts.

Each patient can present with a unique cluster of risk factors that may be relevant in the development of a tendinopathy and for the clinician to decide which to emphasize in assessment and treatment.

Extrinsic factors include excessive volume, magnitude, or speed of loading; training errors such as poor equipment and abrupt or acute changes in amount or type of load (e.g., sudden change to a different shoe type); environmental conditions such as temperature (e.g., cold weather, which makes the tendon stiffer); and ground conditions.

Intrinsic factors include individual biomechanics (malalignments, muscle weakness or imbalance, decreased flexibility), age, and adiposity.

In early-stage disease, inflammation has been demonstrated in peritendinous tissues but is unclear if the inflammation is associated with the etiology of tendinopathy; in end-stage disease, classic inflammatory changes are not frequently seen in tendon pathology in humans [15].

Histologic descriptions of tendinopathies demonstrate degenerative changes and disorganized arrangement of collagen fibers and an increase in vascularity [16].

In the insertional tendinopathies, there are often areas of focal fatty, mucoid, cystic, and hyaline degeneration, calcification, and a change in collagen fiber structure with the loss of the normal parallel bundles [17].

Patients with tendinopathy display a tendon thickening but a reduced energy-storing capacity, meaning that for the same load, their tendons exhibit higher strains than those of healthy individuals.

Furthermore, once symptoms and pain develop, ensuing movement dysfunction may contribute to the chronicity of symptoms. In particular, tendon pain causes widespread motor inhibition in the affected region, evidenced by decreased muscular activity as assessed with electromyography. Individuals with tendinopathy also tend to use movement patterns that place excessive or abnormal load on their tendons; the faulty movement may represent either a root cause or a reason for chronicity or slow resolution [18].

In some cases of chronic tendinopathy, a calcific tendinitis may occur near the insertion of the tendon.

The exact etiology of the origin and of resorption of the calcium deposition is uncertain. Acute calcific tendinitis is largely idiopathic, but some reports suggest that repeated or local trauma is a cause of the calcium deposition, while Uhthoff et al. suggested local hypoxia due to mechanical or vascular change may be the cause. Hypoxia leads to degeneration of tendon substance into fibrocartilage and subsequent calcification, mediated by chondrocyte. The angiogenetic response would allow eventual resorption of the deposit by macrophages, which restores normal perfusion and oxygen tension to the tissue. After resorption of the calcium, the tendon probably regains its original architecture by synthesis of new matrix [19].

Although calcific tendinopathy can occur at the insertion of any tendon, it most commonly affects the shoulder around rotator cuff, Achilles tendon, or patellar tendon. Generally, in the hip area, the calcifications are commonly found in the region of the gluteal tuberosity involving the tendons of the hip abductors. Calcific deposit in the rectus femoris origin is a rare disease first recognized in 1967 by King and Vanderpool, and in recent years, only few cases were reported [20].

Most of the published reports regarding calcific tendinitis of the RF describe involvement of the reflected head; compared to the direct head, calcific tendinitis of the reflected head is more likely to produce an acute episode because of the proximity to the hip capsule. An acute pain exacerbation caused by rupture of calcific material into the joint could be a further eventuality [21].

4.4 Clinical Aspects

RF tendinopathy symptoms include a gradual and progressive onset of pain and tenderness at the anterior aspect of the hip during sport activity which may be reproduced when attempting a straight leg raise or trying to lift the knee up against resistance. Pain and stiffness may be worst in the morning or after periods of rest.

A thorough clinical history and specific physical examination are essential to make the appropriate diagnosis and facilitate a specific treatment plan.

At history, there is often a change in training routine as an increase in mileage, a different training surface, an inadequate warm-up, or stretching program.

Subjectively, the athlete complains of pain when he starts exercising, and typically, the pain is aggravated by exercise, especially during warming up, jumping, and running.

In the cases of acute calcific tendinitis, clinical manifestations include severe localized pain, swelling, tenderness, and loss of function.

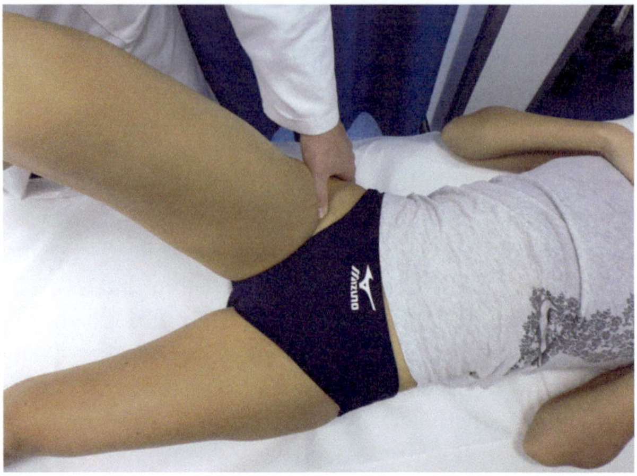

Fig. 4.2 Palpation of the tendon with the hip flexed

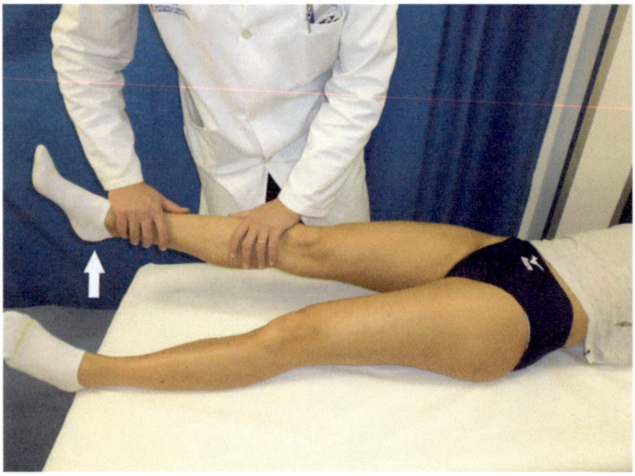

Fig. 4.3 Strength test of the rectus femoris with extended knee

After collecting accurately the clinical history, during physical examination, pain is usually felt by the patient during resisted muscle activation, passive stretching, and direct palpation over the tendon.

Typically, pain could be elicited by palpation and pressure on the tendon: the athlete lies on his back, the examiner is positioned by the affected side bringing the athlete's hip flexed to 90° passively with the knee flexed, and then he pushes on the tendon using as landmark the AIIS (Fig. 4.2).

Strength testing of the rectus femoris should include resistance of hip flexion both with extended and flexed knee (Figs. 4.3 and 4.4). Furthermore, adequate strength testing of the rectus femoris must include resisted knee extension with the hip flexed and extended (Fig. 4.5).

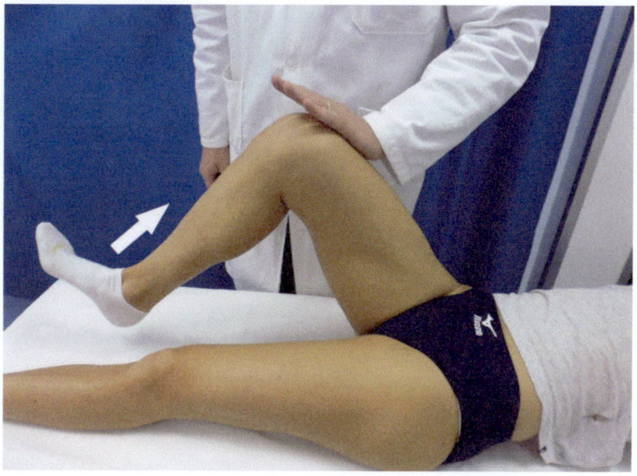

Fig. 4.4 Strength test of the rectus femoris with flexed knee

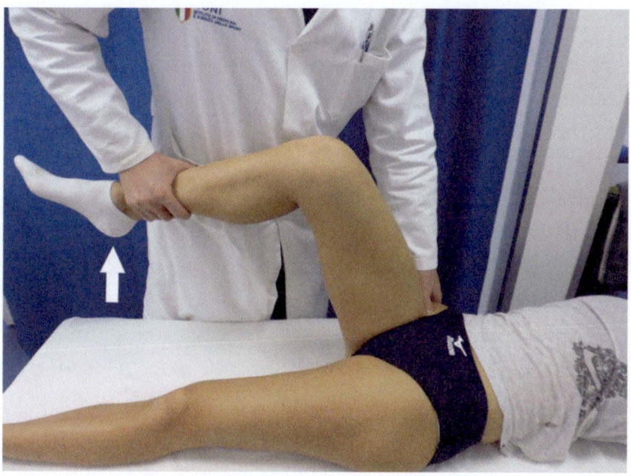

Fig. 4.5 Resisted knee extension with the hip flexed

4.5 Differential Diagnosis

The differential diagnoses are many and often difficult to reach; they must be placed with hip injuries as acute hip joint arthritis, periarticular infections, labral tears, degenerative changes and chondral lesions of acetabulum, stress fractures of femoral neck, and femoroacetabular impingement. During the diagnostic process, another cause of pain which must be kept in mind is the snapping hip. It is a syndrome characterized by pain and recurrent clicks or snaps during active motion of the hip. Three kinds of snapping hips are known: an intraarticular variety (attributable to loose bodies, labral lesions, chondromatosis, joint instability, or ruptured

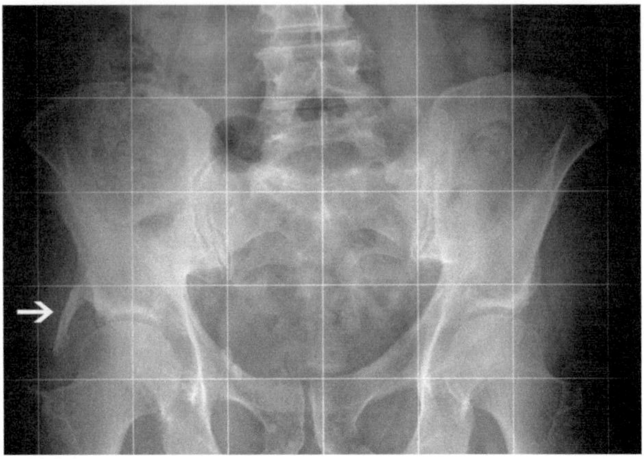

Fig. 4.6 X-ray examination of the pelvis; calcific tendinitis of rectus femoris (*white arrow*)

ligamentum teres), an external extraarticular variety (attributable to subluxation of the posterior aspect of the iliotibial band or the anterior border of the gluteus maximus over the greater trochanter), and an internal extraarticular variety (attributable to subluxation of the iliopsoas or direct RF tendon).

Even if calcific tendinitis of RF direct head is extremely rare, it can impinge against the overlying iliac muscle, resulting in a painful coxa saltans; other pathologic changes involving this tendon could result in similar thickening, potentially predisposing the development of an internal snapping hip [22].

An adequate history and physical examination are the first and the most important steps for a specific diagnosis. In cases of diagnostic uncertainty, advanced imaging techniques such as X-ray examination, ultrasound, or magnetic resonance imaging (MRI) are commonly utilized to assist in diagnosing these diseases.

4.6 Imaging

X-ray examination has only a limited role to play in the diagnosis of rectus femoris abnormalities; AP and slightly oblique view of the pelvis are able to show calcific tendinitis and the presence of major osseous or articular abnormalities (Fig. 4.6).

Tendinopathies can be easily studied with ultrasound and magnetic resonance (MR) imaging, both providing good anatomical details of the tendon and its alterations.

Ultrasonography has been shown to be a noninvasive imaging technique accurate and sensitive in diagnosing tendon injuries in the groin region. It has the advantage of being fast, inexpensive, and widely available, and it can be performed during dynamic tests. Normal findings are readily distinguished from pathological ones providing valuable diagnostic information in association with clinical evaluation, such as location and extent of the injury.

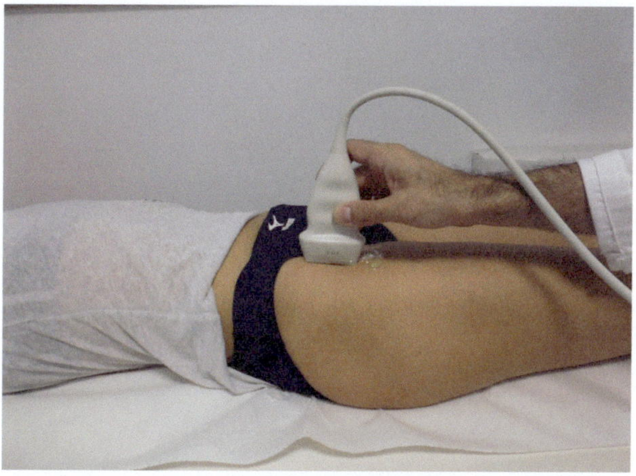

Fig. 4.7 The probe is placed longitudinally on the anterior aspect of the hip

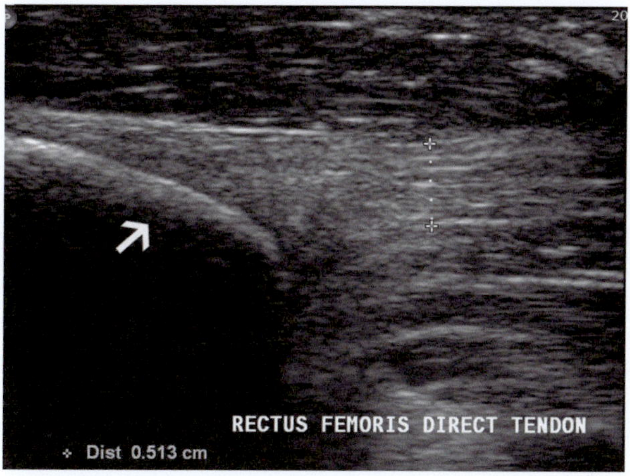

Fig. 4.8 Normal ultrasound longitudinal scan of rectus femoris tendon with a thickness of 0.51 cm at about 10 mm below the anterior inferior iliac spine (*white arrow*)

Rectus femoris direct tendon can be easily appreciated with high frequency transducers using sagittal scans performed taking as anatomical landmark (the AIIS) which can be readily identified by palpation (Fig. 4.7). The transducer is then placed over the anterior aspect of the hip on the axial plane and moved distally for 4–5 cm to visualize the muscle-tendon junction. The direct tendon is then examined with longitudinal scans moving the probe from medially to laterally providing an excellent morphological and structural visualization. In sagittal view the direct tendon is cylindrical with smooth borders, a thickness of about 0.5 cm, and an internal structure homogeneously hyperechoic (Fig. 4.8). On axial scans, the tendon appears as a more or less oval-shaped morphology, located over the AIIS (Fig. 4.9). Sagittal images

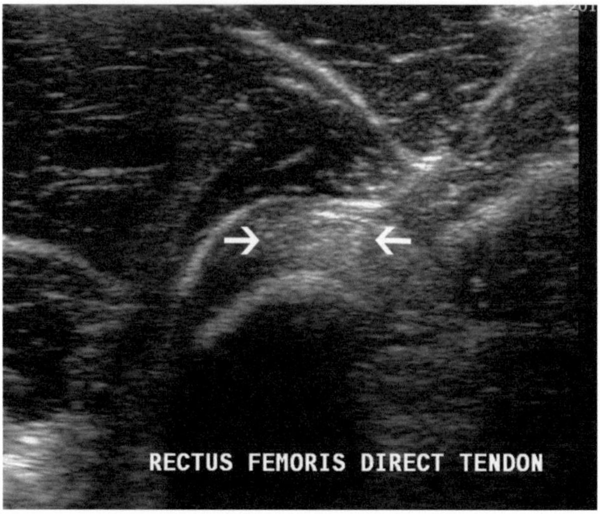

Fig. 4.9 Normal ultrasound axial scan of the tendon (*white arrows*) over the AIIS

allow complete exploration of the direct tendon from its origin at the AIIS to the myoaponeurotic junction. Moving the transducer laterally, the indirect tendon that follows an oblique course appears as a hypoechoic band descending toward the upper rim of the acetabulum, which is best visualized, on oblique axial images [23, 24].

It is known that the pathological modifications caused by overuse on the tendons are represented by changes in the morphology and structure. Pathologic changes may include an irregular, diffuse, or circumscribed fusiform thickening, with or without marked alterations of its structure as the loss of normal fibrillary texture and the presence of variable shape heterogeneously decreased echogenicity areas, corresponding to focal fatty, mucoid, cystic, and hyaline degeneration (Fig. 4.10).

Calcification of the tendon appears as hyperechoic formation of different sizes and shapes with posterior attenuation of the ultrasound beam.

MRI can obtain a tridimensional evaluation imaging, to visualize pathologic conditions of the tendon, clearly depicting all pelvic, hip, and groin changes. MRI is able to provide high intrinsic tissue contrast, which permits the distinction between normal and abnormal tendons, and its high spatial resolution permits detailed anatomic structures to be identified. MRI has superb resolution of the soft tissue structures, does not utilize ionizing radiations, and can aid to diagnose a variety of tendon disorders, representing the investigation of choice in all tendinopathies.

Normal tendons, ligaments, and fibrocartilage have low signal intensity in all sequences.

On the other hand, tendinopathy is characterized by thickening and an increased intrasubstance signal on T2-weighted imaging sequences, which is often the first sign of tendon abnormality. The high–intermediate signal intensity within the

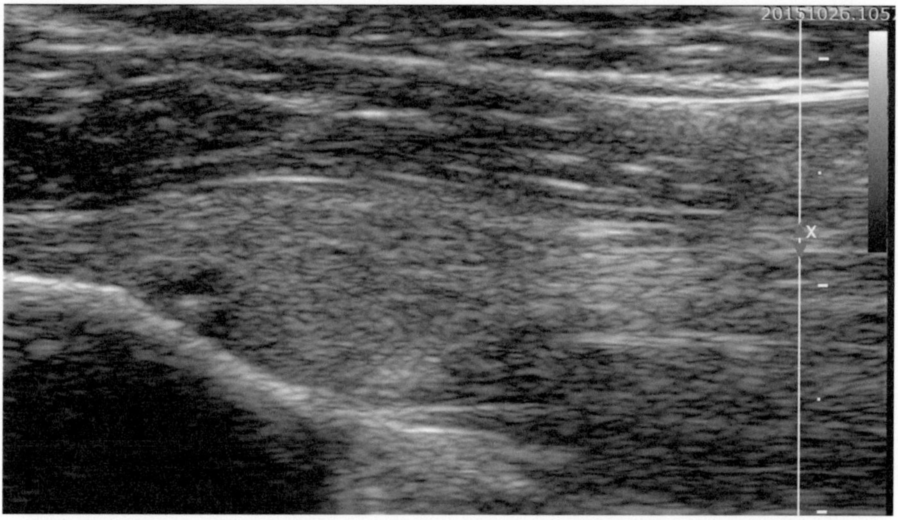

Fig. 4.10 Longitudinal ultrasound scan in rectus femoris tendinopathy; the tendon is thicker with changes in its structure

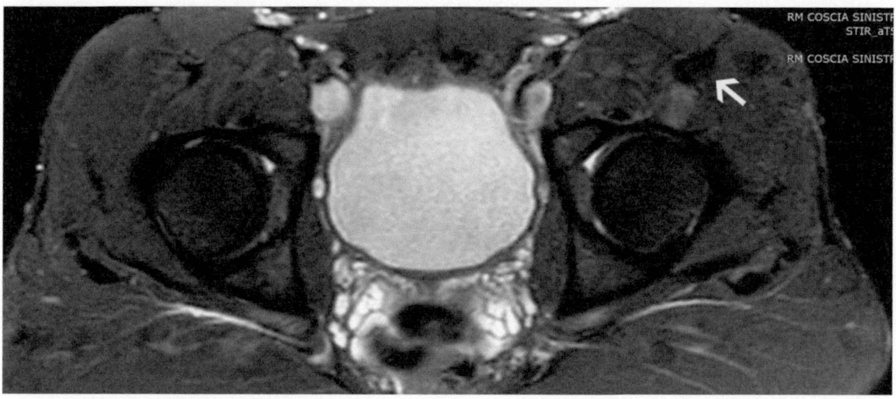

Fig. 4.11 Axial STIR MRI view of the pelvis; the tendon is thicker with minimal internal changes in its structure

substance of the pathologic tendon can be differentiated from fluid, as it appears brighter on T2 sequences.

MRI findings of tendinosis consist of foci of mildly increased signals within the tendon, often longitudinally oriented (Fig. 4.11).

In calcific tendinopathies, MRI shows on conventional spin echo (SE) T1- and T2-weighted images, lower signal intensity in the tendon; however, the calcifications are not always easy to detect with MR imaging.

The most valuable imaging planes are sagittal and axial along the course of the tendon. The coronal images are used when additional information is needed, for example, to see changes at the myotendinous junction and/or at the bone-tendon junction.

It is recommended to acquire images in three planes with the appropriate field of view to include the tendon, the myotendinous junction, and the AIIS proximally.

The use of intravenous contrast is usually not part of the routine examination protocol of rectus femoris tendon as its use adds little in the identification of the lesion.

4.7 Conservative Treatment

Rectus femoris tendinopathy treatment is focused, in early stages, on pain and inflammation reduction, functional restoration, and prevention of reinjuries. Reported treatment strategies for tendinitis vary and mainly comprise conservative management.

Oral nonsteroidal anti-inflammatory drugs (NSAIDs) have been used extensively for decades to treat pain associated with tendon overuse injuries. More recently, the local administration of NSAIDs through gels or patches has been advocated. The evidences suggest both oral and local NSAIDS are effective in relieving the pain associated with tendinopathy in the short term of treatment (7–14 days) [25].

Not surprisingly, the patients who presented with a longer duration and greater severity of symptoms are more likely to have a poor response to both topical and oral NSAIDs.

In addition, long-term NSAID use increases the risk of gastrointestinal, cardiovascular, and renal complications associated with these medications. Overall, a short course of NSAIDs appears a reasonable option for the treatment of acute pain associated with tendon overuse. There is no clear evidence that NSAIDs are effective in the treatment of chronic tendinopathy in the long term.

The therapeutic protocol of rectus femoris tendinopathies should include physical therapy with a wide variety of modalities available in order to draw up a rehabilitation protocol.

First of all, cryotherapy provides acute relief of pain and its use is widely accepted. Repeated applications of melting ice water through a wet towel for 10-min periods are generally effective [26].

Concerning eccentric strengthening programs, they are widely used in rehabilitation; however, this kind of contraction could have a negative effect on the muscle as it is well known that eccentric exercise could cause greater muscle damages to patients than concentric exercise [27]. From these points of views, eccentric exercise should be introduced carefully in the rehabilitation protocols especially in the acute phases and could be performed under supervision at least in the first stages.

Otherwise, the use of manual therapy resulted in an improvement in pain scores and strength. Transverse friction massage has also been used to treat tendinopathy even if a Cochrane review evaluating deep friction massage found no benefit with deep friction massage versus other treatments [28].

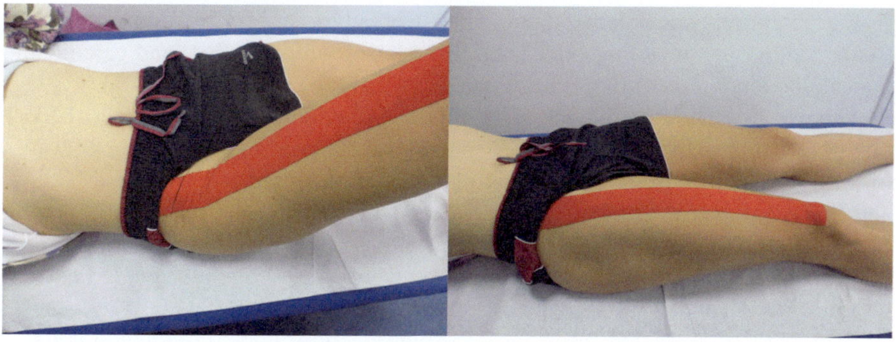

Fig. 4.12 Kinesiotaping in flexed hip (*left*) and in extended hip and knee (*right*)

In some cases a quite new form of tape, called kinesiotaping, could be used. Kinesiotaping has been proved to be effective in various musculoskeletal conditions. Although its precise working mechanism has yet to be fully understood, it is believed to interact with neuromuscular function through mechanoreceptor activation. Kinesiotaping may represent an effective adjunct therapy in the physical rehabilitation program [29] (Fig. 4.12).

Furthermore, other treatment modalities can be applied with good results.

Low-level laser treatment (LLLT) has been studied extensively with mixed results. Some studies showed improvement, treating tendinopathy with LLLT compared to placebo LLLT [30].

Iontophoresis and phonophoresis are noninvasive therapeutic modalities using, respectively, ionizing current and ultrasound, to enhance the delivery of topically applied drugs through the skin; corticosteroids or NSAIDs are commonly used with these modalities to treat tendinopathy, but there is a lack of evidence on their efficacy.

Hyperthermia too has been used in the treatment of tendinopathy but not in the acute phases. This modality involves deep heating machines that combine a superficial cooling system with a microwave-powered heating system. This can increase the temperature of target tissues of approximately 4 °C without damaging the skin. Presumably, this increased temperature results in increased blood flow and subsequent healing to the damaged area. A randomized clinical trial has been published evaluating hyperthermia compared to therapeutic ultrasound in the treatment of tendinopathy demonstrating improvements in pain and patient satisfaction in the hyperthermia group compared to the ultrasound group [31].

Therapeutic ultrasound can be used in the treatment of tendinopathies. A systematic review of physical therapy modalities used for the treatment of shoulder pain suggested ultrasound appeared effective for the treatment of calcific tendonitis [32].

Even though the calcific tendinitis of the rectus femoris is rare and often it may be a self-limited disease, some of the patients do need treatment.

Some authors have reported the use of extracorporeal shock wave therapy (ESWT) with satisfying results [33].

Extracorporeal shock wave therapy has been advocated for treating several soft tissue conditions, including plantar fasciitis, lateral epicondylitis, and calcific and noncalcific tendonitis of the supraspinatus and Achilles tendon.

There is also evidence that tenocytes release growth factors in response to ESWT that may promote tendon healing. Chen et al. reported administering shock waves to a rat Achilles tendinopathy model resulted in increased tenocyte proliferation and increased expression of transforming growth factor-beta 1 and insulin growth factor 1 [34].

Improved efficacy has been demonstrated when using computer-guided navigation in applying shock waves to calcific tendonitis [35].

Eventually, in refracted cases, local steroid injections under computed tomography or fluoroscopic guidance are promising treatment. Local steroid and anesthetic injections are rapid and provide long-standing pain relief and a shortened clinical course, even if the mechanism involved is uncertain.

Eighty milligrams of methylprednisolone in combination with 2 ml of 0.5 % bupivacaine [36] or 40 mg of methylprednisolone with 1.5 cc of lidocaine has been used [37].

Other substances that can be administered by injection in the management of tendinopathies are represented by hyaluronic acid, platelet-rich plasma (PRP), and mesenchymal stem cells (MSC). Regarding the hyaluronic acid, a recent study shows how it could stimulate the synthesis of collagen type I [38]; furthermore Kumai et al. demonstrated how a single injection of high-molecular-weight hyaluronic acid in patients with enthesopathies (lateral epicondylitis, patellar tendinopathy, insertional Achilles tendinopathy, and plantar fasciitis) could be clinically effective [39].

A recent research shows how peritendinous injections of hyaluronic acid could also be used after a single steroid injection [40].

For what concern PRP, several studies underlined its use in tendinopathies. Devenport et al. demonstrate how ultrasound-guided intratendinous injections with PRP could be useful for treatment of proximal hamstring tendinopathy [41].

Furthermore, the majority of preclinical studies in literature show that PRP stimulates the tendon's healing process [42].

Mesenchymal stem cell therapy is a new regenerative approach for treating tendinopathy. For example, treatment of tennis elbow patients with single injection of mesenchymal stem cell showed a significant improvement in short- to medium-term follow-up [43].

In the future, such growth factor- and/or stem cell-based injection therapy can be developed as an alternative conservative treatment for patients with other kinds of tendinopathy such the rectus femoris one, especially in patients that have failed nonoperative treatment before surgical intervention is taken.

Currently, the challenge lies in conducting randomized, controlled clinical trials to determine the essential qualities of these technologies.

4.8 Surgical Treatment

Nowadays in the scientific literature, there are no significant indications on the surgical treatment of RF straight tendon, contrary to what happens to other forms of tendinopathy such as the tendinopathies of the supraspinatus or of the Achilles tendon.

In most cases RF tendinopathy is usually a self-limiting condition, responding well to conservative measures; the majority of patients find adequate relief from conservative treatment, and for this reason, it is not necessary to undergo a surgical intervention. Surgical management could be an effective option in carefully selected patients who have failed 3–6 months of conservative therapy.

Only in the cases of complete rupture of the tendon, surgical repair should be proposed even if there is no definitive treatment protocol to recommend; in fact there are few data published in the literature.

In these cases the tendon stump is inserted via a bony trough prepared in the AIIS, through an anterior (Smith-Petersen) approach, and the sutures are tied over bony tunnels [44].

In painful calcific tendinopathies, arthroscopic excision of tendon calcification yields satisfying results with few risks to the patient, rapid recovery, and satisfactory short-term outcomes.

As stated by Zini et al., it can be removed using a 5.5 mm bur through two standard portals (anterolateral and mid-anterior), after achieving the complete exposure of the calcification [45].

In refractory cases or when a large bone formation occurs after traumatic injuries (i.e., avulsion fracture of AIIS), a surgical excision of the calcification may be necessary, traditionally performed through an anterior approach.

Furthermore, hip arthroscopy gives the chance to treat this pathology providing the opportunity to address concomitant lesions, such as labral tear, femoroacetabular impingement, and cartilage lesions with minimal damage of the soft tissues surrounding the hip area [46].

4.9 Conclusions

Overuse disorders of tendons, bones, and joints represent a widespread problem in sport and a challenge to sports physicians. Even if rectus femoris tendinopathies are not so often observed in the clinical practice of sport medicine, sometimes the strong eccentric loading, like during sprinting and kicking, could lead to a tendinopathy.

Athletes with rectus femoris tendinopathy could refer a gradual and progressive onset of pain and tenderness at the anterior aspect of the hip during sport activity. Pain may be reproduced when attempting a straight leg raise or trying to lift the knee up against resistance. Pain and stiffness may be worse first thing in the morning or after periods of rest.

A thorough clinical history and specific physical examination are essential to make the appropriate diagnosis and facilitate a specific treatment plan. Rectus femoris direct tendon can be easily appreciated with ultrasound using sagittal scans performed taking as anatomical landmark (the AIIS) that can be readily identified by palpation. Chronic conditions could lead to a calcific tendinitis; in this case, clinical manifestations include severe localized pain, swelling, tenderness, and loss of function. In calcific tendinopathies MRI shows on conventional spin echo (SE) T1- and T2-weighted images lower signal intensity in the tendon; however, the calcifications are not always easy to detect with MR imaging; an X-ray could be more appropriate in order to identify a calcification of the tendon.

The differential diagnoses are many and often difficult to reach; a rectus femoris tendinopathy should be distinguished from hip injuries as acute hip joint arthritis, periarticular infections, labral tears, degenerative changes and chondral lesions of acetabulum, stress fractures of femoral neck, and femoroacetabular impingement.

References

1. Lopes AD, Hespanhol Júnior LC, Yeung SS, Costa LO (2012) What are the main running-related musculoskeletal injuries? A systematic review. Sports Med 42(10):891–905
2. Harris-Adamson C, You D, Eisen EA, Goldberg R, Rempel D (2014) The impact of posture on wrist tendinosis among blue-collar workers: the San Francisco study. Hum Factors 56:143–150
3. Orchard J, Seward H (2002) Epidemiology of injuries in the Australian football league, seasons 1997–2000. Br J Sports Med 36(1):39–44
4. Ouellette H, Thomas BJ, Nelson E, Torriani M (2006) MR imaging of rectus femoris origin injuries. Skeletal Radiol 35(9):665–672
5. Rossi F, Dragoni S (2001) Acute avulsion fractures of the pelvis in adolescent competitive athletes: prevalence, location and sports distribution of 203 cases collected. Skeletal Radiol 30(3):127–131
6. Hasselman CT, Best TM, Hughes C 4th, Martinez S, Garrett WE Jr (1995) An explanation for various rectus femoris strain injuries using previously undescribed muscle architecture. Am J Sports Med 23(4):493–499
7. Hapa O, Bedi A, Gursan O, Akar MS, Güvencer M, Havitçioğlu H, Larson CM (2013) Anatomic footprint of the direct head of the rectus femoris origin: cadaveric study and clinical series of hips after arthroscopic anterior inferior iliac spine/subspine decompression. Arthroscopy 29(12):1932–1940
8. Ryan JM, Harris JD, Graham WC, Virk SS, Ellis TJ (2014) Origin of the direct and reflected head of the rectus femoris: an anatomic study. Arthroscopy 30(7):796–802
9. Apostolakos J, Durant TJ, Dwyer CR, Russell RP, Weinreb JH, Alaee F, Beitzel K, McCarthy MB, Cote MP, Mazzocca AD (2014) The enthesis: a review of the tendon-to-bone insertion. Muscles Ligaments Tendons J 4(3):333–342
10. Benjamin M, Kumai T, Milz S, Boszczyk BM, Boszczyk AA, Ralphs JR (2002) The skeletal attachment of tendons – tendon "entheses". Comp Biochem Physiol A Mol Integr Physiol 133(4):931–945
11. Nene A, Mayagoitia R, Veltink P (1999) Assessment of rectus femoris function during initial swing phase. Gait Posture 9(1):1–9
12. Nene A, Byrne C, Hermens H (2004) Is rectus femoris really a part of quadriceps? Assessment of rectus femoris function during gait in able-bodied adults. Gait Posture 20(1):1–13

13. Weinreb JH, Sheth C, Apostolakos J, McCarthy MB, Barden B, Cote MP, Mazzocca AD (2014) Tendon structure, disease, and imaging. Muscles Ligaments Tendons J 4(1):66–73
14. Renstrom P, Woo S (2007) Tendinopathy: a major medical problem in sport. Blackwell Publishing Ltd, Oxford, pp 1–9
15. Cook JL, Khan KM (2007) Etiology of tendinopathy. Blackwell Publishing Ltd, Malden, pp 11–28
16. Khan KM, Cook JL, Bonar F, Harcourt P, Astrom M (1999) Histopathology of common tendinopathies. Sports Med 27(6):393–408
17. Ferretti A (1996) Tendinopatie (Generalità e Classificazione) Casa Editrice Scientifica Internazionale. pp 181–202
18. Scott A, Backman L, Speed C (2015) Tendinopathy-update on pathophysiology. J Orthop Sports Phys Ther 21:1–39
19. Uhthoff HK, Sarkar K, Maynard JA (1976) Calcifying tendinitis: a new concept of its pathogenesis. Clin Orthop Relat Res 118:164–168
20. King JW, Vanderpool DW (1967) Calcific tendonitis of the rectus femoris. Am J Orthop 9(6):110–111
21. Braun-Moscovici Y, Schapira D, Nahir AM (2006) Calcific tendinitis of the rectus femoris. J Clin Rheumatol 12(6):298–300
22. Pierannunzii L, Tramontana F, Gallazzi M (2010) Case report: calcific tendinitis of the rectus femoris: a rare cause of snapping hip. Clin Orthop Relat Res 468(10):2814–2818
23. Bianchi S, Martinoli C, Waser NP, Bianchi-Zamorani MP, Federici E, Fasel J (2002) Central aponeurosis tears of the rectus femoris: sonographic findings. Skeletal Radiol 31:581–586
24. Pasta G, Nanni G, Molini L, Bianchi S (2010) Sonography of the quadriceps muscle: examination technique, normal anatomy, and traumatic lesions. J Ultrasound 13(2):76–84
25. Schorn D (1986) Tenoxicam in soft-tissue rheumatism. S Afr Med J 69(5):301–303
26. Wilson JJ, Best TM (2005) Common overuse tendon problems: a review and recommendations for treatment. Am Fam Physician 72(5):811–818
27. Peake JM, Suzuki K, Wilson G, Hordern M, Nosaka K, Mackinnon L, Coombes JS (2005) Exercise-induced muscle damage, plasma cytokines, and markers of neutrophil activation. Med Sci Sports Exerc 37(5):737–745
28. Brosseau L, Casimiro L, Milne S, Robinson V, Shea B, Tugwell P, Wells G (2002) Deep transverse friction massage for treating tendinitis. Cochrane Database Syst Rev (4):CD003528
29. Paoloni M, Bernetti A, Fratocchi G, Mangone M, Parrinello L, Del Pilar CM, Sesto L, Di Sante L, Santilli V (2011) Kinesio taping applied to lumbar muscles influences clinical and electromyographic characteristics in chronic low back pain patients. Eur J Phys Rehabil Med 47(2):237–244
30. Bjordal JM, Lopes-Martins RA, Iversen VV (2006) A randomized, placebo controlled trial of low level laser therapy for activated Achilles tendinitis with microdialysis measurement of peritendinous prostaglandin E2 concentrations. Br J Sports Med 40:76–80; discussion 76–80
31. Giombini A, Di Cesare A, Casciello G, Sorrenti D, Dragoni S, Gabriele P (2002) Hyperthermia at 434 MHz in the treatment of overuse sport tendinopathies: a randomised controlled clinical trial. Int J Sports Med 23:207–211
32. Philadelphia Panel (2001) Philadelphia panel evidence-based clinical practice guidelines on selected rehabilitation interventions for shoulder pain. Phys Ther 81:1719–1730
33. Oh KJ, Yoon JR, Shin DS, Yang JH (2010) Extracorporeal shock wave therapy for calcific tendinitis at unusual sites around the hip. Orthopedics 33(10):769
34. Chen YJ, Wang CJ, Yang KD, Kuo YR, Huang HC, Huang YT, Sun YC, Wang FS (2004) Extracorporeal shock waves promote healing of collagenase-induced Achilles tendinitis and increase TGF-beta1 and IGF-I expression. J Orthop Res 22:854–861
35. Sabeti-Aschraf M, Dorotka R, Goll A, Trieb K (2005) Extracorporeal shock wave therapy in the treatment of calcific tendinitis of the rotator cuff. Am J Sports Med 33:1365–1368
36. Yun HH, Park JH, Park JW, Lee JW (2009) Calcific tendinitis of the rectus femoris. Orthopedics 32:490

37. Seo YJ, Chang JD, Chang SK, Lee GK (2004) Calcific tendinitis of the rectus femoris. J Korean Orthop Assoc 39:343–346
38. Osti L, Berardocco M, di Giacomo V, Di Bernardo G, Oliva F, Berardi AC (2015) Hyaluronic acid increases tendon derived cell viability and collagen type I expression in vitro: comparative study of four different hyaluronic acid preparations by molecular weight. BMC Musculoskelet Disord 16:284
39. Kumai T, Muneta T, Tsuchiya A, Shiraishi M, Ishizaki Y, Sugimoto K, Samoto N, Isomoto S, Tanaka Y, Takakura Y (2014) The short-term effect after a single injection of high-molecular-weight hyaluronic acid in patients with enthesopathies (lateral epicondylitis, patellar tendinopathy, insertional Achilles tendinopathy, and plantar fasciitis): a preliminary study. J Orthop Sci 19(4):603–611
40. Bernetti A, Mangone M, Paoloni M, Di Sante L, Murgia M, Santilli V (2014) Corticosteroid and hyaluronic acid injection therapy in tennis elbow (lateral epicondylalgia). Med Sport 67(2):289–295
41. Davenport KL, Campos JS, Nguyen J, Saboeiro G, Adler RS, Moley PJ (2015) Ultrasound-guided intratendinous injections with platelet-rich plasma or autologous whole blood for treatment of proximal hamstring tendinopathy: a double-blind randomized controlled trial. J Ultrasound Med 34(8):1455–1463
42. Kaux JF, Drion P, Croisier JL, Crielaard JM (2015) Tendinopathies and platelet-rich plasma (PRP): from pre-clinical experiments to therapeutic use. J Stem Cells Regen Med 11(1):7–17. eCollection 2015
43. Singh A, Gangwar DS, Singh S (2014) Bone marrow injection: a novel treatment for tennis elbow. J Nat Sci Biol Med 5(2):389–391
44. Bottoni CR, D'Alleyrand JCG (2009) Operative treatment of complete rupture of the origination of the rectus femoris. Sports Health 1(6):478–480
45. Zini R, Panascì M, Papalia R, Franceschi F, Vasta S, Denaro V (2014) Rectus femoris tendon calcification. Arthroscopic excision in 6 top amateur athletes. Orthop J Sports Med 2(12):2325967114561585
46. Peng X, Feng Y, Chen G, Yang L (2013) Arthroscopic treatment of chronically painful calcific tendinitis of the rectus femoris. Eur J Med Res 18:49

Chapter 5
Iliopsoas Tendinopathy

Andrea Foglia, Achim Veuhoff, Cesare Bartolucci, Gianni Secchiari, and Gian Nicola Bisciotti

Abstract Iliopsoas tendinopathy represents a 'grey area' in the sports-related biomedical literature, from the terminology used to describe it to its aetiopathogenesis, from conservative management to surgical treatment. Not much has been written about it, and the opinions expressed, despite their being 'evidence based' in some cases, are often conflicting.

In this chapter, the authors review and synthesise information about the different clinical scenarios of iliopsoas tendinopathy.

The authors propose a 'best practice' approach, where daily clinical decisions result from the integration of the health professional's experience, competence and skill with the use of the best available scientific evidence.

A. Foglia (✉)
Sport Rehabilitation Department, Riabilita Clinic, Civitanova Marche, Italy
e-mail: andreafoglia@riabilita.org

A. Veuhoff
Private Practice, Bolzano, Italy

C. Bartolucci
Sport and Internal Medicine, University of Urbino, Urbino, Italy

G. Secchiari
Sport Rehabilitation Department, Riabilita Clinic, Civitanova Marche, Italy
e-mail: segreteria@riabilita.eu

G.N. Bisciotti
Qatar Orthopaedic and Sport Medicine Hospital, FIFA Center of Excellence, Doha, Qatar

G.N. Bisciotti, P. Volpi (eds.), *The Lower Limb Tendinopathies*,
Sports and Traumatology, DOI 10.1007/978-3-319-33234-5_5

5.1 Introduction

Iliopsoas tendinopathy represents a ‘grey area’ in the sports-related biomedical literature. Not much has been written about it, and the opinions expressed, despite their being ‘evidence based’ in some cases, are often conflicting. These discrepancies affect all aspects of the condition: topographic anatomy, functional considerations, nomenclature used, the location of the presumed pathoanatomical changes, aetiopathogenesis and conservative or surgical management.

In this chapter, we shall attempt to propose a ‘best practice’ approach, where daily clinical decisions result from the integration of the health professional’s experience, competence and skill with the conscientious, explicit and judicious use of the best available scientific evidence, combined with the preferences, expectations and needs of the patient/athlete.

5.2 Epidemiology and Aetiopathogenesis

The clinical manifestations affecting the iliopsoas tendon and its associated structures are many and varied. Analysis of the different definitions reported in the literature reveals conflicting descriptions and therefore evident terminological confusion.

Listed below are some of these clinical presentations:

1. Iliopectineal/iliopsoas bursitis and friction bursitis [1, 2].
2. Distal iliopsoas strain with partial or total tendon tears [3].
3. Iliopsoas syndrome, represented by the combination of two different pathophysiological phenomena: iliopectineal bursitis and iliopsoas tendinopathy. The two structures – tendon and bursa – influence each other because of their close proximity [4, 5].
4. Snapping hip syndrome [6–8], which deserves special attention.
   ‘Snapping’ or ‘clunking’ originates from three distinct situations:
   - Intra-articular factors (least common)
   - External factors, i.e. from the iliotibial band (most common)
   - Internal factors

Whereas intra-articular and external problems are *not* related to the *iliopsoas tendon*, internal factors consist of irregularities in its movement: the tendon may meet an obstacle, a hindrance on the iliopectineal eminence, anterior-inferior iliac spine or on the femur head. There may be paralabral cysts acting as an anterior barrier to the passage of the tendon. With regard to the tendon itself, part of the muscle belly may be caught by its own tendon, and there have been reports of a bifid tendon or stenosing tenosynovitis [9, 10]. A snapping phenomenon coming from the iliopsoas tendon is also considered to represent the true ‘snapping hip’ [11].

A snapping hip produced by the iliopsoas tendon does not necessarily cause pain or require treatment.

Leaving aside the topic of strain with partial or complete tear of the muscle-tendon complex, usually the outcome of a particularly violent event, we will deal with the remaining causes of tendinopathy: snapping related to iliopsoas bursitis. A further remark about the connection between the bursa and the tendon, a structure whose integrity has been damaged by long-lasting inflammatory processes, will be more susceptible to inciting events.

Turning to the risk factors and mechanisms of injury, a crucial passage in identifying the aetiology is obtaining information about two variables [12]. Risk factors are classified into intrinsic and extrinsic, modifiable and non-modifiable. A few *intrinsic risk factors*, which are predominantly non-modifiable (or poorly modifiable), can be identified for iliopsoas tendon disorders: age between 15 and 40 years; female sex (predominant in the reported series); hip hypermobility [13]; coxa vara, a bony crest above the lesser trochanter (very rare); previous strains; previous surgical procedures that have modified the mechanical axis of the lower limb; and caused exuberant scar tissue in the area of passage [14, 15]. In hypermobile subjects the periarticular muscular structures have to work more intensely to control the excess of movement [13]. As regards strength (a factor closely related to neuromuscular control), instead, reduced capacity of the gluteal musculature, combined with hypermobility, could constitute a further risk factor for the development of iliopsoas tendinopathy [13].

5.3 Clinical Examination

In the physical examination, the examiner's ability to distinguish between 'normal' (clinically irrelevant and not related to the athlete's reported complaint) and abnormal (clinically relevant and potentially related to the patient's clinical condition) is crucial. Through the physical examination, the examiner aims to:

- Appreciate and recognise '*relevant clinical signs*'.
- Relate the clinical signs to the athlete's reported symptoms.

Possible signs and symptoms during palpation are:

- Pain on passive, active or active-resisted hip flexion
- Pain on internal rotation or with passive hyperextension
- Tenderness to palpation over the femoral triangle

Another aspect to be considered is hypermobility on account of its role as an intrinsic risk factor. Hypermobility is evaluated with the Beighton score or with the questionnaire developed by Hakim and Grahame [16].

We believe it useful to suggest specific manoeuvres for internal snapping hip and a checklist with additional items that may lend support to a suspicion of bursitis. At the same time, however, given their doubtful diagnostic power, these tests should be taken as merely provocative tests to help orient the diagnosis.

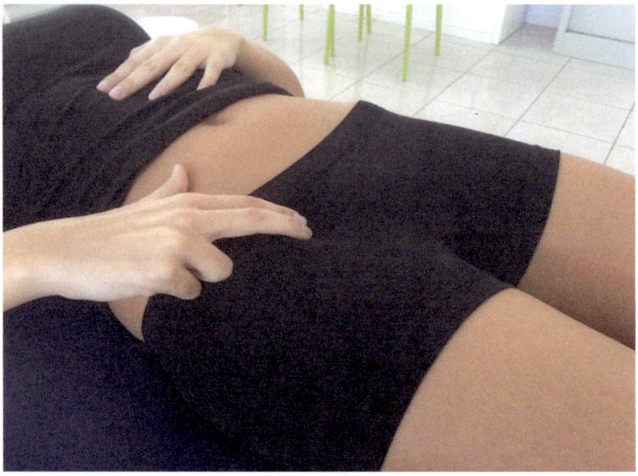

Fig. 5.1 An important point is to ask to the patient to point the area where the snapping is felt

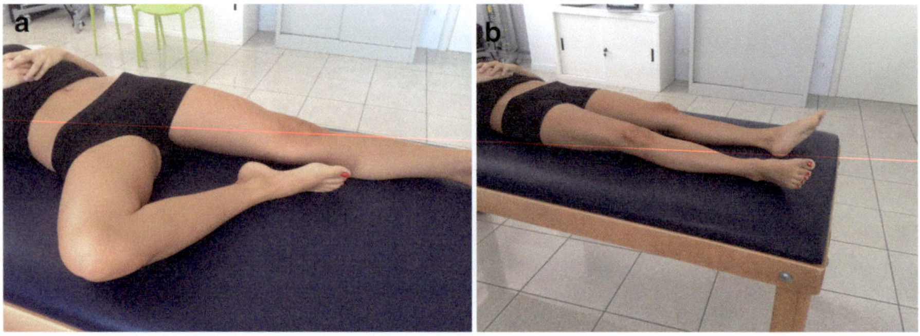

Fig. 5.2 (**a**, **b**) When we ask to the patient if he/she can reproduce the snapping, an audible snap and/or palpable snap is considered as a positive test

It is important to ask to the patient to point the area where the snapping is felt (Fig. 5.1) and ask the patient if he/she can reproduce the snapping. As stated, the snapping can often be reproduced only by the subjects themselves, who are used to the combination of movements required to produce it. After these two primary steps, the snapping might also be induced passively. This is a manoeuvre for eliciting internal hip snapping.

The dynamic manoeuvre needed to elicit the snap phenomenon may vary considerably within the affected population. Also different is the starting position: the patient may be seated, standing or lying down. Among all these variables, there is one constant: the passage from flexion to extension. An audible snap and/or palpable snap is considered a positive test (Fig. 5.2). The snapping can often be eliminated or significantly lessened by applying pressure over the iliopsoas tendon.

Byrd invites us not to interpret the snapping phenomenon as an intra-articular problem, stating that the medical history combined with the physical examination is the most valuable instrument available to the clinician. Snapping of the iliotibial band (external cause), very similar in pain and sound produced, is easier to differentiate from articular injury because of its lateral location [14]. Three more interesting tests to assess iliopsoas disorder are shown in Figs. 5.3, 5.4 and 5.5.

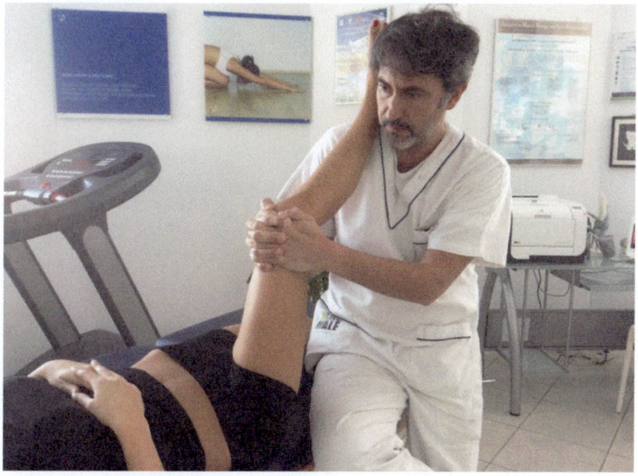

Fig. 5.3 Functional muscle testing of the iliopsoas muscle the subject lies supine. The test leg is flexed maximally in the hip and knee joint. The examiner tries to extend the flexed hip by pulling it with two hands wrapped around the femur just proximal to the knee. Pain is recorded as 'yes' or 'no'. Strength is assessed by the examiner as 'strong', 'intermediate' or 'weak'

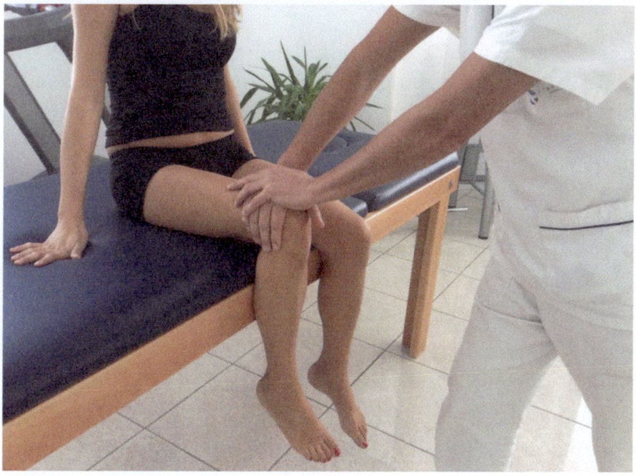

Fig. 5.4 Iliopsoas-related pain or iliopsoas weakness may be also exacerbated by testing hip flexion strength while the patient is seated. The same items (pain and strength) will be investigated and recorded

The previously mentioned 'psoas syndrome', on the other hand, consists of the simultaneous presence of an internal snapping hip and an iliopectineal bursitis [15]. As regards 'symptomatic' snapping phenomenon, once the clinician has considered the athlete's clinical history, the symptoms elicited by the provocation tests and the snapping reproduced by the procedure reported above, the diagnosis can be considered probable.

5.4 Imaging in Iliopsoas Tendinopathy

The presence of numerous, often coexisting, anatomical and mechanical factors predisposing to the development of similar signs and symptoms, coupled with the difficulty discriminating between external and internal factors on the basis of the patient's medical history and clinical examination, calls for an integration with imaging techniques to help establish the diagnosis. In the presence of the

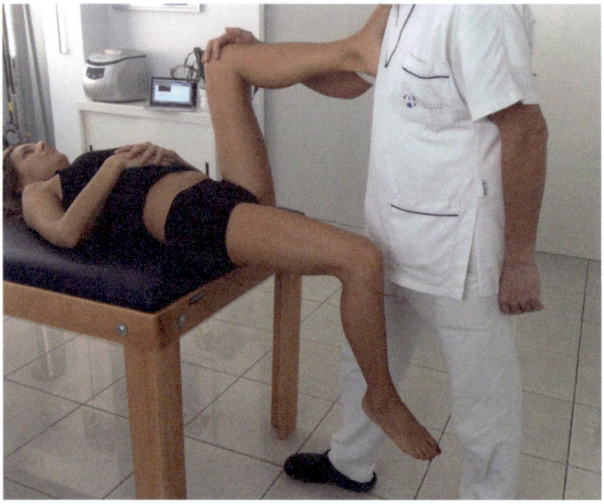

Fig. 5.5 Modified Thomas Test. When the patient holds their knee to their chest, the following thing should become immediately apparent: if the psoas is of normal length, then the dependent thigh should be free to hang down 45° below the plane of the table. In this picture, the patient's right psoas is significantly shortened. A positive Thomas test can also be an indicator of damage to the bursa, which leads to our next point. Bursitis of the iliopectineal bursa (of the iliopsoas) may be suspected if items from the following checklist are added [17, 18]

'*pathognomonic*' signs and symptoms of a snapping hip syndrome, obtained from the medical history and physical examination, ultrasound proves to be a frequently useful, rapid, economically sustainable, first-choice procedure for the static and dynamic study of the iliopsoas tendon and related tendinous structures [19]. A dynamic ultrasound study allows assessment of the function of the tendon along its entire course: the examiner can therefore identify possible 'obstacles' and appreciate the resulting abnormalities in tendon movement [20] with considerable discriminatory precision [21]. In brief, ultrasound can help to detect, characterise and stage iliopsoas tendinopathy.

The particular topographical location of the iliopsoas tendon requires the use of sonographic probes of varying frequency, ranging between 3.5 and 18 MHz [9]. The advantages and disadvantages of ultrasound imaging in general also apply to the study of the iliopsoas muscle. Advantages include its noninvasiveness, the absence of ionising radiation, widespread availability and the possibility of performing scans also during muscle contraction. Disadvantages are selective imaging documentation and operator dependence.

In order to identify the iliopsoas tendon, two scanning planes are commonly used. The first is a transverse/oblique plane along the iliopubic line [9]. The second is a pure transverse plane passing below the first plane, just beneath the anteroinferior iliac spine [9].

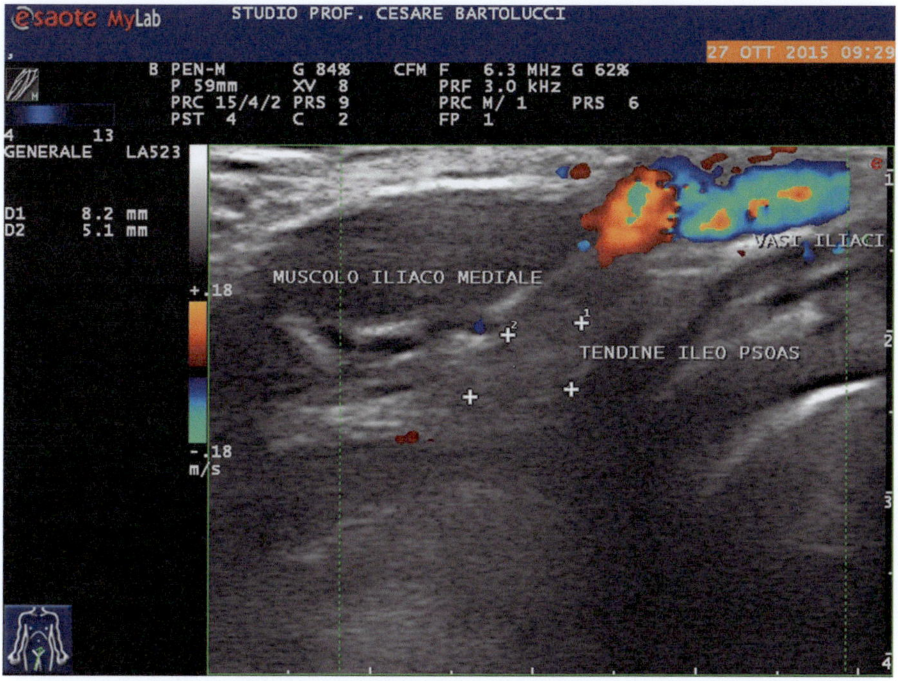

Fig. 5.6 Sonographic view of iliopsoas tendon

The field of view of the first scanning plane, with an axial oblique section above the anteroinferior iliac spine, includes the lateral and medial portion of the iliac muscle (separated by the intramuscular fascia of the iliac muscle), the superior pubic ramus, the iliopubic eminence and the femoral vessels, which can be optimally studied with the aid of colour Doppler imaging [22, 23]. The iliopsoas tendon can be distinguished below the femoral vessels and the lateral and medial fascia of the iliac muscle (Fig. 5.6).

The field of view of the second scanning plane, with a transverse section below the anteroinferior iliac spine, includes the sartorius muscle, the rectus femoris, the infratrochanteric portion of the iliac muscle and the medial and lateral portions of the iliac muscle with their intramuscular fascia. The iliopsoas tendon can be distinguished in contact with the acetabular rim (Fig. 5.7).

On ultrasound, it is sometimes possible to detect the rare anatomical variant of a bifid tendon [24–26]. Partial or complete divisions have also been reported that are not depicted by ultrasound but can be seen on magnetic resonance imaging (MRI).

Before insertion of the tendon on the posterior aspect of the lesser trochanter, a synovial bursa is visualised. The bursa is only seen when it contains fluid. The iliopsoas bursa is an area of natural expansion of the hip joint cavity. Bursal distension is commonly seen in trauma; in inflammatory, infectious or

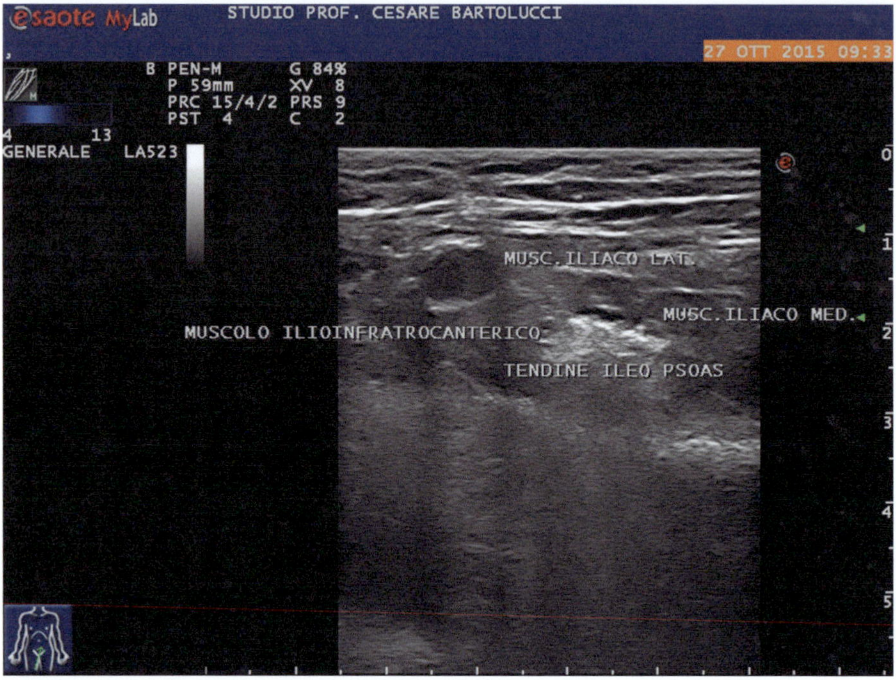

Fig. 5.7 Sonographic view of iliopsoas tendon in contact with the acetabular rim

degenerative arthritis; in villonodular synovitis; and in overuse and impingement syndromes [27].

Ultrasound has a significant role in the differential diagnosis between a large bursal distension and an inguinal or pelvic mass such as lymphadenopathies, hernias or tumours [22].

MRI is successfully used to obtain well-defined images of the overdistended iliopectineal bursa [2, 28], of the components of the iliopsoas muscle and its musculotendinous continuum. In the distal portion, close to the insertion on the lesser trochanter, MRI allows detection of possible tendon avulsion. Completion of the assessment with MRI allows differentiation between tumours and other types of lesions.

The various causes of iliopsoas bursitis include those secondary to femoral pathology such as avascular necrosis of the femoral head. In particular, MRI is used in distal tendon tears in elderly patients with avulsion of the insertion on the lesser trochanter [29, 30]. The anatomy of the iliopsoas tendon is in fact fairly complex, especially at its insertion on the lesser trochanter, where fibres also arrive directly from the lateral portion of the iliac muscle as well as from a very thin tendon separated from the iliopsoas by a thin cleft of fat. Even in iliopsoas tendinopathies affecting endurance athletes, MRI proves to be superior to ultrasound in the differential diagnosis of inguinal pain which may be produced by partial tears or tears involving only a few fibres.

5.5 Conservative Treatment of Iliopsoas Tendinopathy

Snapping hip syndrome in general (internal or external) may be treated conservatively in a similar manner to other tendinopathies: by suspension, reduction or modification of athletic activity or any other activity that causes pain, application of physical agents (ice), oral administration of drugs (NSAIDs) [31], local injection of NSAIDs or corticosteroids [32, 33] – even though this last approach is poorly supported by scientific evidence [34, 35] – and not better specified 'sports rehabilitation' [14, 15, 36].

As regards manual therapy for the iliopsoas muscle-tendon complex, and in particular transverse friction massage, we believe that this technique is unlikely to be effective. Deep transverse friction massage administered to other more superficial, and thus more accessible, anatomical structures and in similar pathoanatomical settings has not been shown to modify clinically relevant outcomes [37].

The most commonly described exercises for the treatment of tendinopathies are eccentric exercises. In *eccentric* contraction, the tension generated is sufficient to exceed the external load on the muscle, and the muscle fibres lengthen despite there being a contraction.

Although this type of contraction has been used for many years, its mechanism of action on both the micro- and macrostructure of the tendon and on pain reduction has yet to be elucidated [38]. As regards the loading dose, speed of execution, number of series and repetitions of an exercise, there is currently no consensus or a high level of evidence or strength of the recommendations, as these parameters are still being studied.

In addition to these *general* indications, the literature offers no other proven therapeutic solutions for the clinical presentations discussed in this chapter. We will briefly mention the medical treatment of iliopsoas bursitis.

Treatment of iliopsoas bursitis differs depending on the severity of the clinical presentation and the presence of possible complications. If the bursitis is mild, it is usually sufficient to apply an ice pack, observe a period of rest (absolute or relative) and administer an anti-inflammatory agent to reduce inflammation and pain. In some cases, however, it may be necessary to aspirate the liquid contained in the inflamed bursa (ultrasound-guided aspiration) and sometimes inject corticosteroids and/or anaesthetic directly into the bursa so as to resolve the inflammation and reduce the risk of recurrence. In addition to using drugs to control inflammation and pain, the treatment of bursitis may also include application of local physical therapies (such as cryotherapy) [39].

There is good evidence of the clinical effectiveness of *conservative medical treatment* in the presence both of bursitis and of iliopsoas tendinopathy (evidence level 1a/1b).

The literature indicates that the conservative medical treatment for the two structures is very similar [40].

In the presence of pathological conditions affecting the tendon and its associated structures, multimodal interventions are generally adopted: therapeutic exercise associated with manual therapy (e.g. transverse friction massage, Cyriax), instrumental therapy (ultrasound, shockwave, low-level laser, iontophoresis with NSAIDs) and the use of taping [41]. Much of the literature on the subject consists of expert opinion with the lowest level of evidence.

Further research is needed to find out which treatment strategy combined with therapeutic exercise will provide the best results in the rehabilitation of tendinopathy in general [41].

5.6 Surgical Treatment of Iliopsoas Tendinopathy

Surgical treatment represents the last resort for resolving the patient's symptoms and is used when conservative treatment has failed. With regard to the iliopsoas bursa, various surgical procedures have been proposed: a plain bursectomy or a capsulectomy to gain access to the bursa in the case of bursitis not responding to conservative treatment. Another frequently used procedure is arthroscopic synovectomy, the surgical removal of a portion of the synovial membrane, combined, in selected cases, with iliopsoas tendon release (see below) [40, 42]. Review of the literature on the subject has revealed a fair level of evidence.

For snapping hip syndromes in general, the surgical approach consists in resecting, lengthening and/or relaxing the involved tight tendon, in order to reduce the impingement and eliminate the symptomatic snapping. The surgical approach comprises several possible procedures depending on the cause of the snapping hip syndrome [14, 43, 44].

For external causes, various types of iliotibial tract resections may be performed. For each type of operation, different approaches exist (e.g. iliotibial tract resections may be partial, Z shaped or elliptical shaped), and to date no significant differences in terms of clinical outcome have been found among the various techniques proposed.

For the less common intra-articular disorders, on the other hand, the primary causes may be very different: there may be partial tears of the acetabular labrum, synovial osteochondromatosis or loose bodies inside the joint (e.g. from osteochondral fractures) [43, 45]. The surgical approaches will vary based on the specific diagnosis.

For internal causes the tendon of the iliopsoas muscle may be lengthened [46], or a complete arthroscopic release may be performed. Endoscopic release provides good results, also supported by midterm follow-up [47].

Surgical reduction of the tendon diameter is compensated for by a regeneration of '*tendinous*' tissue over an average period of 20 months: the tendon diameter returns to 80 % of its initial value. In current endoscopic resection techniques, surgeons try to preserve a ratio of 60 % muscle to 40 % muscle tendon in the remaining tissue, and it is very likely that the preserved continuity of muscle fibres provided by this procedure prevents retraction of the tendon ends, thereby contributing to partial regeneration. In addition to the regrowth, the iliopsoas muscle fibres continue to run parallel to the iliopsoas tendon, and after the operation this bundle of remaining muscle fibres will insert directly onto the femur without a tendon, thereby contributing to overall strength which some authors believe is fully restored (to presurgery levels).

5.7 Conclusions

Iliopsoas tendinopathy remains a poorly investigated subject characterised by many grey areas. There is no consensus in the literature on the terminology used, and there are no experimental studies of good methodological quality. Moreover, the number of epidemiological studies (aetiological, observational, cohort studies, etc.) is insufficient to enable the precise identification of risk factors. Finally, there is a lack of valid and reliable diagnostic tests to be combined with imaging to be able to establish a firm diagnosis. All this translates into clear limitations for our study and our clinical practice, and in particular, the inability to derive significant data from the publications available today for our reference models [48, 49].

References

1. Forstner R et al (1998) Sonographic diagnosis of iliopectineal bursitis – a contribution to the differential diagnosis of leg-swelling. Fortschritte auf dem Gebiet der Röntgenstrahlen und der neuen bildgebenden Verfahren 169(4):408–411
2. Wunderbaldinger P, Bremer C, Schellenberger E et al (2002) Imaging features of iliopsoas bursitis. Eur J Radiol 12:409–415
3. Bui KL, Ilaslan H, Recht M, Sundaram M (2008) Iliopsoas injury: an MRI study of patterns and prevalence correlated with clinical findings. Skeletal Radiol 37(3):245–249
4. Saiko S, Stuber K (2009) Psoas major: a case report and review of its anatomy, biomechanics, and clinical implications. J Can Chiropr Assoc 53(4):311
5. Tufo A, Gautam JD, Cox WJ (2012) Psoas syndrome: a frequently missed diagnosis. J Am Osteopath Assoc 112(8):528
6. Guillin R, Cardinal E, Bureau NJ (2009) Sonographic anatomy and dynamic study of the normal iliopsoas musculotendinous junction. Eur J Radiol 19:995–1001
7. Winston P, Awan R, Cassicy JD et al (2007) Clinical examination and ultrasound of self-reported snapping hip syndrome in elite ballet dancers. Am J Sports Med 35:118–126
8. Konczak CR, Ames R (2005) Relief of internal snapping hip syndrome in a marathon runner after chiropractic treatment. J Manipulative Physiol Ther 28(1):67
9. Bancroft LW, Blankenbaker DG (2010) Imaging of the tendons about the pelvis. AJR Am J Roentgenol 195(3):605
10. Alpert JM, Kozanek M, Kelly BT. Three-dimensional anatomical relationship of the iliopsoas and acetabular labrum. Presented in occasion of the 55th Annual Meeting of the Orthopaedic Research Society
11. Kendra S et al (2013) MR appearance and clinical significance of changes in the hip muscles and iliopsoas tendon after arthroscopic iliopsoas tenotomy in symptomatic patients. HSS J 9:236–241

12. Bahr R, Krosshaug T (2005) Understanding injury mechanisms: a key component of preventing injuries in sport. Br J Sports Med 39(6):324–329
13. Day H et al (2011) Hypermobility and dance: a review. Int J Sports Med 32(7):485–489
14. Byrd JW (2005) Snapping hip. Oper Tech Sports Med 13:46–54
15. Idjadi J, Meislin R (2004) Symptomatic snapping hip: targeted treatment for maximum pain relief. Phys Sportsmed 32(1):25–31
16. Hakim AJ, Grahame R (2003) A simple questionnaire to detect hypermobility: an adjunct to the assessment of patients with diffuse musculoskeletal pain. Int J Clin Pract 57:163–166
17. Wyss J, Patel A (2013) Therapeutic programs for musculoskeletal disorders. Demos Medical Publishing, New York. ISBN 13 978-1-93628-740-6
18. Noesberger B, Eichenberger AR (1997) Overuse injuries of the hip and snapping hip syndrome. Oper Tech Sports Med 5(3):138–142
19. Hashimoto BE, Green TM, Wiitala L (1997) Ultrasonographic diagnosis of hip snapping related to iliopsoas tendon. J Ultrasound Med 16:433–435
20. Deslandes M, Guillin R, Cardinal E, Hobden R, Bureau NJ (2008) The snapping iliopsoas tendon: new mechanism using dynamic sonography. Am J Roentgenol 190:576–581
21. Choi YS, Lee SM et al (2002) Dynamic sonography of external snapping hip syndrome. J Ultrasound Med 21:753
22. Bancroft LW, Blankenbaker DG (2010) Imaging of the tendons about the pelvis. AJR Am J Roentgenol 195(3):606
23. Newman JS, Adler RS, Bude RO, Rubin JM (1994) Detection of soft-tissue hyperemia: value of power Doppler sonography. Am J Roentgenol 163:385–389
24. Guilin G, Cardinal C, Bureau JN (2009) Sonographic anatomy and dynamic study of the normal iliopsoas musculotendinous junction. Eur J Radiol 19:999
25. Tatu L, Parratte B, Vuillier F, Diop M, Monnier G (2001) Descriptive anatomy of the femoral portion of the iliopsoas muscle: anatomical basis of anterior snapping of the hip. J Radiol Anat 23:371–374
26. Philippon MJ, Devitt BM, Campbell KJ, Michalski MP, Espinoza C, Wijdicks CA (2014) LAPRADE: anatomic variance of the iliopsoas tendon. Am J Sports Med 42(4):807–811
27. Di Sante L, Paoloni M et al (2014) Groin pain iliopsoas bursitis: always a cause-effect relationship? J Back Musculoskelet Rehabil 27(1):103–106
28. Zameer H, Hunjun J, Choudur HN (2011) Imaging of the bursae. J Clini Imag Sci 1(1):6
29. Bancroft LW, Blankenbaker DG (2010) Imaging of the tendons about the pelvis. AJR Am J Roentgenol 195(3):608
30. Piggott RP, Doody O, Quinlan JF (2015) Iliopsoas tendon rupture: a new differential for atraumatic groin pain post-total hip arthroplasty. BMJ Case Rep 2:32
31. Bancroft LW, Blankenbaker DG (2010) Imaging of the tendons about the pelvis. AJR Am J Roentgenol 195(3):607
32. Garala K, Power RA (2013) Iliopsoas tendon reformation after Psoas tendon release. Case Rep Orthop 2:1–4
33. Reich M, Shannon C, Tsai E, Salata MJ (2013) Hip arthroscopy for extra-articular hip disease. Curr Rev Musculoskelet Med 6(3):250–257
34. Frizziero A, Trainito S et al (2014) The role of eccentric exercise in sport injuries rehabilitation. Br Med Bull 110(1):47–75
35. Mehallo CJ, Drezner JA, Bytomski JR (2006) Practical management: nonsteroidal anti-inflammatory drug (NSAID) use in athletic injuries. Clin J Sports Med 16(2):170–174
36. Whal CJ, Warren RF, Adler RS, Hannafin JA, Hasen B (2004) Internal coxa saltans (snapping hip) as a result of overtraining: a report of 3 cases in professional athletes with a review of causes and the role of ultrasound in early diagnosis and management. Am J Sports Med 32(5):1302–1309
37. Loew LM, Brosseau L, Tugwell P, et al. (2014) Deep transverse friction massage for treating lateral elbow or lateral knee tendinitis. Cochrane Database Syst Rev (11):CD003528

38. Murtaugh B, Ihm JM (2013) Eccentric training for the treatment of tendinopathies. Curr Sports Med Rep 12:175–182
39. Grainger AJ, Rowbotham EL (2011) Ultrasound-guided intervention around the hip joint: musculoskeletal imaging – review. Am J Roentgenol 197(1):122–127
40. Johnston CAM, Wiley JP, Lindsay DM, Wisemand DA (1998) Iliopsoas bursitis and tendinitis: a review. J Sports Med 25(4):271–283
41. Dimitrios S (2015) Exercise for tendinopathy. World J Methodol 5(2):51–54
42. Gilliland WR, Murphey MD, Papadoupolos PJ, Zembrzuska H (2012) Iliopsoas bursitis. J Musculoskelet Med 3:53–54
43. Bond RP, Snyckers CH (2010) Management of sports overuse injuries of the lower limb: an evidence-based review of the literature. SA Orthopaedic J 9(2):48–58
44. Anderson SA, Keene JS (2008) Results of arthroscopic iliopsoas tendon release in competitive recreational athletes. Am J Sports Med 36:2363–2371
45. Randelli F et al (2012) Intra-articular loose body removal during hip arthroscopy. Orthopedics 3(7):476
46. Jacobson T, Allen WC (1990) Surgical correction of the snapping iliopsoas tendon. Am J Sports Med 18(5):470–474
47. Ilizaliturri VM et al (2005) Internal snapping hip syndrome: treatment by endoscopic release of the iliopsoas tendon. J Arthroscopic Related Surg 21(11):1375–1380
48. Van Mechelen W, Hlobil H, Kemper HC; op cit
49. Meeuwisse WH; op. cit

Chapter 6
Quadriceps Tendinopathy

Stefano Respizzi, M.C. d'Agostino, E. Tibalt, and L. Castagnetti

Abstract The quadriceps can be considered a relative strong structure of the extensor apparatus of the knee; nevertheless, it can be affected and weakened by degenerative changes, under the influence of local and systemic factors. In some cases, progression of tendinopathy can lead also to spontaneous, partial, or complete rupture. For this reason, prevention and treatment of predisposing factors, as well as early recognition, objective grading, and monitoring of structural alterations, can be helpful in identifying those ones more susceptible to rupture. Symptomatic enthesopathy is rarely the unique cause of bilateral simultaneous and complete rupture of the quadriceps.

Quadriceps tendon tear is a not so common injury, usually occurring in patients older than 40 years of age, frequently due to a fall during sudden quadriceps muscle contraction. Early recognition of this injury can be strategic to ensure a more rapid healing, as well as a better recovery and prognosis.

For complete quadriceps tendon rupture, surgery is the treatment of choice, while in partial tears, an accurate assessment of the degree of the lesion and disability, or loss of function, can aid the clinician in deciding surgical versus conservative treatment. Conservative treatment of partial tears of the quadriceps tendon consists in a full extension brace for 6 weeks, followed by a protected range of motion exercises, that can guarantee a good outcome and regain of function in the follow-up. When surgical treatment is required, 6 weeks of postoperative immobilization with intense rehabilitation are indicated, for obtaining the best functional outcomes as well.

All grades of tendinosis are usually treated conservatively as first-line therapy. Among conservative treatments, biophysical stimulations (extracorporeal shock waves and some so-called physical therapies), as well as autologous growth factors, surely represent some innovative, safe, and effective therapeutic strategies that are

S. Respizzi (✉) • M.C. d'Agostino • E. Tibalt • L. Castagnetti
Dipartimento di Medicina Fisica e Riabilitazione Funzionale, Humanitas Research Hospital, Via Manzoni 56, Rozzano, Milan 20089, Italy
e-mail: stefano.respizzi@humanitas.it

G.N. Bisciotti, P. Volpi (eds.), *The Lower Limb Tendinopathies*, Sports and Traumatology, DOI 10.1007/978-3-319-33234-5_6

indicated in conjunction with rehabilitative programs, in order to obtain, besides anti-inflammatory and analgesic effects, a positive action on tendon tissue and its remodeling processes, for improving recovery.

6.1 Etiopathogenesis and Clinics

Quadriceps tendon injuries include a spectrum of diseases, ranging from tendinosis to partial-thickness tears to complete tendon rupture. Relatively uncommon, between the injuries of the knee, nevertheless they can be considered the second most common ones, after patellar fracture [1]. Moreover, in clinical practice, quadriceps enthesopathy is less common than the patellar one [2].

It has been described in the literature also the possibility of a "calcific tendonitis" of the quadriceps, although an uncommon condition. It has to be considered, in any case, not a "benign" condition, and an awareness of this tendinopathy and the potential complication of quadriceps tendon damage are important, when investigating acute symptoms associated with the extensor mechanism of the knee [3].

Quadriceps tendinopathy has been described to be more frequent in the elderly population, practicing regular sports activities, as well as in weight lifters, due to the fact that the quadriceps tendon is particularly subjected to load, especially in the deep squat [4].

In the older patient population, quadriceps tendon tears usually occur in the setting of a slip and fall. In most of the cases, there are preexisting degenerative changes within the tendon, thought to be due to degeneration or repetitive microtrauma. In younger patients, acute tears are usually sports related, due to sudden acceleration forces or extreme stress [1].

From a general point of view, it manifests with pain along the top of the knee; also it shows resistance during contraction of the quadriceps [4].

Extensor mechanism disruptions of the knee are relatively uncommon but serious injuries. They are clinically diagnosed by the triad of swelling around the knee, palpable defect, and inability to perform straight leg raise. According to Kumar et al., the most common form of disruption would be patellar fracture, followed by rupture of the patellar tendon and the quadriceps tendon. A simultaneous rupture of a patellar tendon and the opposite quadriceps tendon is extremely rare, and different mechanical, systemic, and local factors are involved. The quadriceps rupture is more common in older subjects (>50 years) with associated systemic factors, such as obesity, gout, and local degenerative changes [5].

According to Hardy et al., the predictive value of a spur for rupture of the quadriceps tendon should be considered, in the light of the obvious selection bias of their cohort of patients chosen for operative repair. Although the prevalence of a patellar spur in the normal population is unknown, nevertheless it is as uncommon as rupture of the quadriceps tendon. Thus, the presence of a radiographically identified spur should alert the examining doctor, to the possibility of such an injury in patients with traumatic failure of the extensor mechanism [6].

Bilateral traumatic ruptures of extensor tendons are being increasingly reported, and it is important to consider a bilateral pathology, in all those cases presenting with traumatic rupture on one side. The commonest cause of bilateral simultaneous rupture would appear to be a sudden violent contraction of the quadriceps mechanism, with the knees slightly flexed and feet firmly planted on the ground. It is important to feel for tenderness and defects in both the suprapatellar and infrapatellar regions, as both ruptures can occur simultaneously in spite of having two different pathogeneses [5].

As already mentioned, chronic tendinopathy may evolve in many cases toward progressive tendon degeneration, with possible rupture. This type of injury is usually the consequence of a forced contraction of the quadriceps, with the knee flexed and the foot fixed to the ground, but the pathogenesis has to be considered as multifactorial, as correlated with some general disorders like renal insufficiency (especially with hemodialysis substitutive therapy), primary or secondary hyperparathyroidism, and some other conditions, which impair and weaken the osteotendinous junction [2, 7–10].

Other comorbidities that may cause spontaneous rupture are represented by diabetes, rheumatoid arthritis, and gout, use of quinolones, corticosteroid injections, anabolic steroids, statins, and obesity [8–10]. According to some of the authors, there would be also a genetical predisposition, especially when bilateral rupture of the quadriceps tendon occurs [11]. From a general point of view, some histopathological changes of tendon structure (as abnormal collagen distribution and increased production of type III collagen fibers by tenocytes) seem to be correlated with spontaneous rupture, generally due to minor trauma [8].

Classically, the quadriceps tendon rupture frequently occurs in the attempt to recover balance, in order to avoid a fall. A considerable tension on the tendon occurs, when there is an important eccentric contraction of the quadriceps femoris and the knee is in a half-bent position.

Pain, loss of extension, and suprapatellar gap are the clinical signs of the quadriceps tendon rupture. The clinical assessment can be difficult in this case, due to tenderness and swelling, that increase the risk of missed diagnoses and/or diagnostic delay [9].

Extensor mechanism ruptures might be easily overlooked and misdiagnosed, and delayed diagnosis of quadriceps tendon rupture is not so rare. In these cases, the literature recommends early surgical repair within 72 h [12].

Patients suffering from this injury complain of a painful and swollen knee. They are unable to walk without some sort of assistance and usually hold their leg as straight as possible. Despite these clinical signs, misdiagnosis is frequent, ranging from 39 to 67 %. A gap in the tendon may not be convincingly palpable, and the patient's ability to raise his/her leg straight with the use of the medial and lateral patellar retinaculum or iliotibial band may convince the inexperienced observer that only a few fibers of the tendon have been ruptured. However, the results of the repair may be compromised if the delay to surgery exceeds a few days and no clinical diagnostic test has been described to date [12]. The high rate of misdiagnosis did not decrease with the introduction of ultrasound and MRI investigations. In addition, these instrumental investigations can be considered costly and time consuming in an emergency department. The reasons for delayed diagnosis are probably multifactorial, and the consequences can be considered important, as the outcome could be severely affected [12].

Inspired by the O'Brien test for complete rupture of the Achilles tendon, Jolles et al. proposed in the literature a new minimally invasive test that directly can determine the integrity of the quadriceps tendon in its five distal centimeters [12].

With the patient lying in the supine position, in aseptic condition, a 25-gauge needle is inserted at a right angle through the skin of the thigh, at a midline point, 5 cm proximal to the superior border of the patella. The needle is inserted gently through the skin until further resistance is felt, so that the needle's tip is just within the substance of the quadriceps tendon but without transfixing it. A passive knee flexion and extension movement is then performed, and the movement of the hub of the needle is observed. Two distinct types of response may occur. One response (negative test) is swiveling of the needle about its pivot point in the skin which indicates that the tendon is intact throughout its distal 5 cm. If no swiveling of the needle is observed (positive test), this indicates loss of continuity of the extensor apparatus (quadriceps tendon between its insertion and the position of the needle) [12].

Only few cases of bilateral simultaneous complete quadriceps rupture, in patients with symptomatic enthesopathy, have been previously reported. Arumilli et al. stressed the importance of warning patients of the risk of developing complete tendon rupture, when they present with an enthesopathy around the knee [13].

6.2 Imaging

Although many cases of quadriceps rupture can be diagnosed clinically, partial tendon tears may be more difficult to assess clinically, as some degree of function can be maintained in any case. When tendon tears are acute, soft tissue swelling and associated hematoma may obscure the tendon defect on physical examination and may limit the clinical evaluation. With delayed presentation of a tear, the tendon defect may not be evident due to scar tissue formation. There may also be partial return of quadriceps function after several weeks, with the risk of confusing the diagnosis [1].

Therefore, accurate imaging can aid diagnosis and directly affect patient treatment. Radiographs are usually not diagnostic for quadriceps tendon tear. The use of magnetic resonance imaging for the diagnosis of quadriceps tendon tears has been advocated, but its accuracy has not been defined. Bianchi et al. described the usefulness of sonography for complete quadriceps tendon tears with surgical correlation [1].

6.2.1 *Quadriceps Tendinopathy*

In normal conditions, the quadriceps tendon is visible at ultrasound examination with anechogenic and "multistratus" appearance, in relation to the presence of 2–4 tissue layers. The most frequent anatomical situation is the presence of three layers: the more superficial stratus comes from the more distal part of the rectus femoris, the deeper one derives from the front fascia of the vastus intermedius, and the intermediate one directly from the fascia between the three vastus muscles (intermedius, lateralis, and medialis) [14]. The quadriceps tendon has an area of major weakness, at its distal end, and it is described as the area where tendinopathies arise more frequently. Moreover, in clinical practice, it is possible to observe occasionally some small changes of tendon structure, even in asymptomatic subjects [15].

The ultrasound images of quadriceps tendinopathy can be extremely heterogeneous, from some degenerative alterations limited to a single layer to larger ones engaging the whole tendon. In the first case, tendinopathy can be recognized as a hypoechoic oval image, while in the second one, a wider hypoechogenicity of the different collagen layers will be described, together with thickening of the different layers and loosening of the fibrillar structure, as pathognomonic signs of degenerative tendon disease [15].

Frequent etiologies of quadriceps tendinopathy can be represented by a chronic overload, related to professional activity or overweight, as well as seronegative spondyloarthropathies [15]. In all these conditions, it is possible to demonstrate, through ultrasound examination, the presence of calcifications. Moreover, in seronegative spondylopathy, some areas of bony erosion and soft tissue swelling can be detected, while in calcific overload, enthesopathy calcifications on the tendon surface or in the intermediate layers may be visible [16].

Generally, when a localized tenderness and thickening along the course of the tendon are clinically visible, under sonographic examination, they correspond to a hypoechoic area and pathologic hypervascularization phenomenon. This ultrasound picture, as already mentioned, is sometimes present even in asymptomatic individuals. Some of the authors emphasize that the presence of echographic and structural alterations, in the absence of symptoms, could represent a risk factor for the development of painful symptoms in the future [17].

6.2.2 Tendon Injuries

The obliteration of the "quadriceps shadow," the presence of a mass in the suprapatellar soft tissues secondary to tendon retraction, and the avulsion of a bony segment from the proximal pole of the patella are all typical radiographic features. Another feature that can be considered as suggestive of quadriceps tendon rupture is the so-called "low-riding" patella or patella baja. By the ratio between the length of the patellar tendon and the length of the patella in the lateral projection, it is possible to calculate the index of Insall–Salvati, which is useful for identifying a low patella, if the value is lower than zero [18].

Compared to traditional radiography, ultrasound examination is a more effective method for diagnosing the rupture of the quadriceps tendon [10]. Foley et al. studied the ability of sonography in detecting those quadriceps tendon tears that require surgical treatment (high-grade partial tears and complete ruptures). After having examined 239 consecutive sonographic cases, they were able to demonstrate that sonography is an effective tool for identifying quadriceps tendon tears requiring surgical treatment (high-grade partial tears and complete ruptures) [19].

Magnetic resonance imaging (MRI) is another important instrumental method for tendon evaluation, especially in case of injury. Some main different situations can be described. In case of partial rupture, at least one of the layers is still intact. The superficial layer is the most common site of injury, followed by the intermediate one [20]. In this case, the size of the lesion does not increase with distal end traction of the patella. Finally, we must consider that if the peritendinous envelope is intact, the diagnosis may be difficult. When a total breakage occurred, there is an interruption of all the tendon layers, with a possible hematoma in the area of the lesion. By the traction of the patella, it is possible to observe an increase in the interval between the two tendon stumps. The framework of MRI in complete breaking of the quadriceps tendon demonstrates a retracted proximal stump and a wavy look of the patellar tendon, caused by the lack of tensile force applied to it [2].

Already in 1994, Bianchi S. et al. confirmed that sonography should be considered in the diagnostic workup and treatment planning of patients with suspected tears of the quadriceps tendon, for evaluating quadriceps tendon rupture, due to its noninvasiveness and high degree of sensitivity and specificity [21]. In the following years, ultrasound has been extensively used as a diagnostic tool before surgery, for diagnosing acute traumatic tears of the patellar and quadriceps tendons; these ones are rare injuries, requiring immediate repair to reestablish knee extensor continuity and allow early motion. More recently, Swamy et al. concluded that ultrasonography is not a reliable method in establishing the diagnosis of acute injuries to the extensor mechanism of the knee, especially for the quadriceps tendon ruptures in obese and very muscular patients. When a certain clinical ambiguity is present, MRI scan is a recommended investigation tool, to be taken before any surgical treatment [22].

6.3 Conservative Treatment

The conservative therapeutic approaches to quadriceps tendinopathy are various, and among them, some programs of physiokinesitherapy can be considered, besides manual medicine and different manipulative approaches on soft tissues. From a general point of view, quadriceps tendinopathy is responsive to physiotherapeutic treatments, according to the same general principles of patellar tendinopathy [23]. Abnormal fascial tensions of the thigh frequently hesitate in an uncoordinated contraction of the quadriceps that ultimately hesitates in tendinopathy of the extensor apparatus of the knee. For this reason, an effective approach, in terms of tenderness reduction, can be obtained by treating the fascia of the quadriceps femoris [24].

Eccentric exercises, as much as for some other tendinopathies, play surely a key role also in the conservative and rehabilitative treatment of quadriceps tendinopathy. Even for those tendons subjected to autologous growth factor (platelet-rich plasma or PRP) injections, the need for a standardized rehabilitative program is emphasized, based on a progressive submaximal eccentric work [25].

Dimitrios et al. in 2012 demonstrated that the combination of eccentric training and quadriceps static stretching exercises would be superior to eccentric training alone, in order to reduce pain and improve function, both at the end of treatment and at the end of follow-up as well [26]. Nevertheless, sometimes, the eccentric work can be more painful to be completed; moreover, if performed during the competitive season, it has, in addition to worsening pain, poorer immediate benefits, resulting in poor adhesion to the rehabilitative program [27]. A more immediate effect in controlling pain relief in tendinopathies seems to be obtainable by isometric exercises, with sustained effect for at least 45 min, as well as by an increase in quadriceps strength, through increased voluntary isometric contraction [28].

Setting a timely and proper rehabilitation treatment is also very crucial after surgery, along with the need of a protected load. The rehabilitation program will be developed with exercises aimed to recover range of motion and strengthen the quadriceps. Patients who undergo delayed repair are at risk for a compromised result, due to loss of full knee flexion and decreased quadriceps strength, although a functional extensor mechanism is likely to be reestablished [29].

Many studies demonstrated that treatment involving eccentric training can be effective in the conservative management of chronic tendinosis, although the mechanisms of action are still under study. In particular, Kubo et al. in 11 healthy volunteers were able to demonstrate some changes in blood circulation of the Achilles tendon, during and after repeated eccentric contractions, being more remarkable than those during and after repeated concentric ones [30].

From a general point of view, intact tendons adapt slowly to changes in mechanical loading, whereas in healing tendons, the effect of mechanical loading or its absence is dramatic. Numerous animal studies show that immobilization of healing tendon compromises the healing process [31–33], and many other studies show that tendons adapt to changes in mechanical loading [34]. Nevertheless, some authors hypothesized and demonstrated that tendon tissue would have a "memory" of loading episodes, thus allowing short loadings being enough to elicit improved healing, while suggesting that patients might be allowed early short loading episodes, following a tendon lesion, in order to obtain a better outcome [35]. However, some details about amplitude, frequency, and duration of mechanical stimulation are still partly unknown, as well as the appropriate time point during the repair process to start loading and how to avoid overload. Furthermore, in animal models as well as in humans, there is a great individual variation in tendon response to mechanical stimulation [35].

Moreover, tendon healing/recovering is a complex and highly regulated process that is initiated, sustained, and eventually concluded by a large number and variety of molecules. Growth factors represent one of the most important classes of molecular families involved in tendon healing, and many studies have elucidated their functions, especially in more recent years [36].

Nowadays, the use of PRP has become increasingly popular in tendon and muscle repair. The scientific rationale for its application is based on the fact that it contains a wide variety of growth factors as insulin-like growth factor 1 (IGF-1), transforming growth factor β (TGFβ), vascular endothelial growth factor (VEGF), platelet-derived growth factor (PDGF), and basic fibroblast growth factor (bFGF), and also in vivo, at the site of a tendon injury, platelets are activated and release their factors [37].

Although in the last years the use of PRP in clinical practice is increasing, literature concerning PRP applications is still under debate. In any case, many studies already demonstrated that PRP use for tendon repair can have a positive effect, probably due to an enhancement of the reparative processes. For these reasons, it can be taken into consideration in case of chronic tendinopathy not responsive to conservative treatment [38].

From a general point of view, tendinopathy can be considered as the failure of a chronic healing response, associated with both chronic overloaded or unloaded states. Although several conservative therapeutic options have been proposed in the literature, very few of them are supported by randomized controlled trials. The use of injectable substances such as PRP, autologous blood, polidocanol, and corticosteroids in and around tendons is not supported by strong clinical evidence. Further randomized controlled trials are necessary to define the best conservative management of tendinopathy [39].

If, nowadays, therapeutical exercise represents one of the most important strategic approaches for tendinopathies, nevertheless, some biophysical regenerative therapies can be applied successfully, in order to reduce inflammation and pain and to positively interfere with a local altered turnover of tendon tissue. From this point of view, it has been recently underlined, for example, the efficacy of laser therapy in the field of tendinopathies, despite the need for more studies about this topic. The mechanisms of action would seem related to reduction of inflammation and increased collagen synthesis [40].

Among *biophysical therapies*, nowadays, extracorporeal shock wave therapy represents a valid tool for treating tendinopathies, including quadriceps tendinopathy, while considering this specific anatomic region as part of the extensor compartment of the knee, for which this mechanotherapy has been already demonstrated to be a valid tool. Interestingly, when applied in the musculoskeletal and, in general, in non-urological fields, ESWT has no pure mechanical effect of disruption, but a real biological action on cells and tissues (due to mechanotransduction), with a success rate, according to the literature, up to 91 % (for jumper's knee, Achilles tendinitis, plantar fasciitis, rotator cuff "tendinitis," and greater trochanter pain syndrome) [41–44]. More in details, some clinical experiences would indicate this therapy as effective in treating tendon pathologies, especially when some other conservative treatments have failed, although the mechanisms of action remain still under study [41–43, 45, 46].

From the experimental point of view, tendon and tenocytes have been extensively studied in the field of shock wave (SW) mechanobiology. Some of the authors described, for example, that an optimal SW treatment would promote the healing of a "collagenase" – Achilles tendinitis – by inducing TGF-beta1 and IGF-1 secretion, with the effect of reducing edema, swelling, and inflammatory cell infiltration in experimentally injured tendons. Moreover, in this condition, the authors were able to demonstrate an intensive tenocyte proliferation and progressive tendon tissue regeneration, related to the expression of cell nuclear antigen (PCNA), besides intensive

TGF-beta1 and IGF-1 expression, quite similar to what happens in the early stage of tendon healing. On the basis of these results, it has been hypothesized that physical SW stimulation could increase the mitogenic responses of tendons [47].

Moreover, in the literature, there are many other evidences of a possible direct action of SW on tendon cells, thus implying also a possible future involvement in tendon healing and regenerative therapies. These effects can be so summarized [48–54]:

1. Increased expression of lubricin
2. In vitro enhancing of functional activities of ruptured tendon-derived tenocytes (proliferation and migration)
3. Ehancement of cell vitality and proliferation, besides expression of typical tendon markers and anti-inflammatory cytokines
4. Reduced expression of several metalloproteinases and interleukins (MMPs and ILs)

Regarding the effects of SW on tendons, very recently the biochemical responses of tendons after SW stimulation have been described by microdialysis, in humans; moreover, it was hypothesized that this type of mechanical stimulation could be able to improve tendon remodeling in tendinopathies, by promoting the inflammatory and catabolic processes, that are associated with removal of "pathological" matrix constituents, thus suggesting a potential scientific background for future studies and clinical applications [54].

6.4 Surgical Treatment

From a general point of view, in complete quadriceps tendon rupture, surgery is indicated, whereas tendinosis is usually treated conservatively. According to the extension of the tear and the resulting loss of function, partial tears may be treated surgically [3, 55]. Accurate assessment of the degree of partial tears and the degree of disability can aid the clinician, in determining surgical versus conservative treatment [1]. Conservative treatment of partial tears of the quadriceps tendon consists in a full extension brace for 6 weeks, followed by a protected range of motion exercises, allowing good outcomes and regain of function [3].

Biomechanical studies have demonstrated that normal quadriceps tendon, if subjected to longitudinal tensional strength, can withstand loads up to 30 kg/mm before going to meet at break. It is also estimated that it needs a force equal to three times the body weight, resulting in a fall in knee flexion and maximal contraction of the quadriceps muscle, to lead a tendon rupture. According to what is described, it is understandable that quadriceps tendon tear is an uncommon injury. Nevertheless, the most common modality of rupture is a minor trauma (such as a simple fall or an eccentric contraction of the quadriceps muscle), and usually it represents the end stage of a long process of chronic degeneration and overuse [55, 56]. As already mentioned, in most of the cases, rupture is a spontaneous event, sometimes bilateral, and occurs preferably in older patients, especially if affected by metabolic diseases [57]. Structural tendon alterations are related to muscle atrophy and tendon structure degeneration, but also to modification of the microcirculation. Rupture often occurs in those tendons suffering from fatty, cystic, or myxoid degeneration or characterized by the deposition of calcium salts; all these conditions can modify the tendon architecture and, consequently, its biochemical properties and resistance capacity [58–61]. It has also been suggested that the presence of a patellar spur, a bony prominence at the quadriceps tendon insertion point of the proximal pole, may be related to the rupture itself [62]. Rarely ruptures occur in high-level athletes, and they usually result from an eccentric load on the extensor mechanism. Unfortunately, prodromal symptoms and predisposing factors are almost always absent, and even respecting timing and surgical procedure, a low rate of return to play is described [63, 64]. In athletic population, in contrast with the older ones, a different process involving repetitive microtrauma is thought to occur in the quadriceps tendon, which can be subclinical and eventually lead to tendon ruptures. Ipsilateral tendinopathy of the extensor apparatus may be found in patients who subsequently suffer a quadriceps tendon tear [58]. There are also some iatrogenic conditions (such as total knee replacement, lateral release, and steroid injections) that can modify the normal structure of the quadriceps tendon, with the risk of tendon rupture [55]. The most common rupture site of the quadriceps tendon is located between 1 and 2 cm from the superior pole of the patella, while, in older people, rupture most probably occurs at the osteotendinous junction. This area is less vascularized, thus suggesting that a vascular imbalance may contribute to the pathogenesis of the rupture itself [55]. The vascular supply to the quadriceps tendon is usually sustained by three systems: the medial arcade (that supplies the medial border of the tendon), the lateral arcade (that supplies the lateral border), and the peripatellar vascular ring [59]. In relation to the vascular supply of the quadriceps tendon, some authors proposed that the articular side of the tendon, the deepest one, may be exposed to a relative compressive strength, produced by the bone femoral condyles, thus involving an impairment of the vascular supply [59]. From a general point of view, the viscoelastic properties of the tendon lead fairly quickly to a retraction after rupture, thus making it necessary to proceed surgically as soon as possible, in order to avoid pathological muscle retraction and fibrosis [55–57, 60, 64].

The most widely accepted method for repairing the quadriceps tendon when an acute rupture occurs is the *primary suture repair*, consisting in continuous interlocking sutures, passed through the distal end of the tendon and then secured through some drill holes made into the patella. Regarding the transosseous technique, it is usually used a drill to create a small groove in the upper pole of the patella, whereas tendon sutures are passed through the tendon with Krackow, Kessler, or an equivalent technique. Regarding the transosseous technique, it is usually used a drill to create some small grooves in the upper pole of the patella, whereas tendon sutures are passed through the tendon with Krackow, Kessler, or an equivalent technique. In this way, strong transosseous sutures are placed through the patella, thus securing the distal part of the quadriceps tendon to bone [60, 64, 65].

In the literature, a variety of reinforcement techniques have been described, in order to add an extra support to the primary repairs. These techniques are especially useful, and in case of poor quality of the tendon tissue, or if retraction of torn ends is present, they include wire augmentation, autografts, allografts, and synthetic materials. With all recent advances in technology, numerous studies describe the use of suture anchors for fixation of the quadriceps tendon [66]. This technique can be performed with a smaller incision while preventing potential violation of the patella – tendon junction. Moreover, as another advantage, pilot holes for anchor placement are not transosseous, thus decreasing the potential complication of patella loosening [67, 68]. Human cadaveric studies demonstrate that quadriceps tendon repair with suture anchors yields significantly better biomechanical results than transosseous sutures. These data support a more consistent load-to-failure strength and allow an early partial weight bearing, immediately after surgery. With respect to traditional, primary transosseous technique, there is a much higher cost [69]. Sooner after surgery, the knee is protected with a brace that holds the joint in an extended position for a time varying from 2 to 6 weeks, before starting with progressive knee flexion exercises, according to the surgical technique [70].

Delayed quadriceps tendon rupture requires some more complex surgical techniques, such as the *Scuderi* and *Codivilla* techniques. The *Scuderi* technique consists of a direct repair of the quadriceps tear, reinforced by a tendon partial-thickness triangular flap, turned down and sutured on the superficial aspect of the patella. Nevertheless, the Codivilla method, if presence of significant retraction of quadriceps, can be used: a full-thickness inverted-V-shaped incision is made in the tendon. The base of tissue triangle obtained in the tendon can be moved distally to allow the tear to be approximated and repaired. The proximal aspect of the inverted V can be then repaired side to side and the remaining flap turned down and used as augmentation [56].

Complications are relatively uncommon and include deep venous thrombosis or pulmonary embolism, heterotopic ossifications, superficial and deep infection, and reruptures. Quadriceps muscular atrophy and muscular strength deficit can be present in most of the cases, but generally this does not have any influence on the satisfaction of the patient. No significant differences in order to final results among the surgical techniques used in primary repair are reported, as generally, functional and clinical outcomes seem to be very good; on the contrary, a delay in surgical repair can have an adverse influence on the outcome [56].

Over the years, the repair techniques have progressed from simple suture with catgut or silk to wire-reinforced repair, pullout suture fixation through the patella, suture anchor fixation, tendon lengthening repair, Scuderi technique, allograft, autograft, and synthetic materials. Recently, some authors reported their results using arthroscopy [71]. The purpose of reporting spontaneous quadriceps tendon rupture cases was to describe a new surgical procedure using arthroscopy, which indicated the positive effect of stable fixation followed by early range of motion exercise on the result of treatment [71]. Many investigators reported that the shorter the period between injury and surgery, the better will be the clinical outcome, regardless of surgery method, age, or body mass index (BMI), in patients with quadriceps tendon with no underlying diseases. Delayed diagnosis leads to unsatisfactory clinical outcomes; early diagnosis and early restoration of function are important for preventing disability [71].

Regarding postoperative rehabilitation, it has been reported that prolonged knee immobilization for 6–8 weeks after primary suture was necessary to allow complete healing of the repair and to ensure an acceptable outcome. In addition, postoperative rehabilitation should be determined according to the presence of the underlying diseases, influence of body weight, and period between injury and surgery, and surgical methods with arthroscopic repair of quadriceps tendon rupture can provide excellent results [71].

Adequate repair of the quadriceps and patellar tendons to the patella is essential for a functional extensor mechanism. Too often, these injuries are missed as a result of inadequate suspicion of lesion or confusion with other potential knee injuries. A careful examination, combined with imaging, can detect these injuries, which should be repaired promptly, if the patient is a suitable surgical candidate, in order to provide the most optimal outcomes. In the case of delayed presentation, retraction of the quadriceps tendon yields a challenging reconstruction problem, often requiring the use of allograft and advanced reconstruction techniques, with less predictable results. Every effort should be made to avoid missing this diagnosis [72].

6.5 Synthesis and Therapeutic Indications

Quadriceps tendon is a very strong structure contributing to the extensor mechanism of the knee. The structural and biomechanical properties of the quadriceps tendon allow it to sustain very high loads without rupture. Nevertheless, it can be affected and weakened by degenerative changes, due to some local and systemic factors, although less frequently than some other anatomic districts. Many degenerative age-related changes of the tendon tissue have been described, such as fatty and myxoid degeneration, tendon fibrosis, decrease in quantity, and change in type and cross-links of collagen fibers, microangioblastic dysplasia, and calcifications [73]. Several clinical conditions have been reported to induce tendon degenerative changes: for example, renal diseases, long period of hemodialysis, and uremia are associated with spontaneous tendon rupture, affecting maturation of collagen and quadriceps muscle fiber atrophy [74]. In addition, hyperparathyroidism causes dystrophic calcifications and subperiosteal bone resorption and can weaken the osteotendinous junction between the quadriceps tendon and patella [74]. Diabetes mellitus has also been reported to cause fibrinous necrosis and vascular damage, as observed in quadriceps tendon rupture specimens [73]. Other metabolic and rheumatic diseases such as gout, pseudogout, rheumatoid arthritis, systemic lupus erythematosus, obesity, and steroid intake have been reported to induce tendon degenerative changes [74].

Progression of tendinopathy can lead in some cases to spontaneous partial or complete rupture. For this reason, early recognition and preventing of predisposing factors, as well as objective grading and monitoring of quadriceps structural alterations, will be helpful in identifying those ones most at risk of rupture. Symptomatic enthesopathy can be a rare and unique cause of bilateral simultaneous complete quadriceps rupture [13].

From a general point of view, quadriceps tendinopathy treatment is mainly conservative, and it is based on rehabilitation, biophysical therapies, and autologous growth factors (PRP). Among biophysical therapies, nowadays, those ones which seem to induce greater therapeutic efficacy on degenerative tendon pathology can be considered laser and extracorporeal shock wave therapy (ESWT) [40, 43]. ESWT represents a new therapeutic frontier, by its ability not only to induce an anti-inflammatory effect but also a possible trophic effect on tendon remodeling as well [43].

Rehabilitation is an important basis for functional recovery of quadriceps tendon, and it is based on the general principles applied to patellar tendinopathy [23–28, 30].

The use of innovative techniques such as PRP represents an interesting method, although current studies are not yet fully explaining, while requiring further scientific and clinical trials [36–39].

The tendon tissue response to load consists of three phases: linear deformation, elastic deformation, and plastic deformation. The first one depends only on flattening of the crimp pattern of collagen fibers (2 % of the strain), the second one is due its behavior to intramolecular sliding of collagen triple helices in which the fibers become aligned in parallel fashion (4 % of the strain), and the third one is characterized by a plastic deformation and a microscopic failure of tissue. Approximately at 10 % of strain, macroscopic failure arises. Sudden and eccentric contractions of quadriceps, as occurring during a fall in attempt to maintain balance, can exceed the phase of plastic deformity and may lead to an incomplete or complete rupture [75].

Quadriceps tendon tear is a not so common and often misunderstood injury, usually occurring in patients older than 40 years of age, due to a fall with sudden quadriceps muscle contraction. The earlier the injury is diagnosed right away, the better the prognosis will be. Surgical treatment is required, and at least 6 weeks of postoperative immobilization with intense rehabilitation are needed to obtain the best functional outcomes [76].

The viscoelastic properties of tendons and muscles determine the degree of retraction during the rupture process. Unless the original length is restored, the retracted quadriceps become too short to function properly, and, as demonstrated in neglected ruptures, only inadequate muscle function can be expected. Furthermore, early motion and tensile stresses appear to promote the organization and remodeling of collagen fibers, decrease scar tissue, and increase strength [76].

Surgical techniques for quadriceps tendon repair are different. Generally, for mid-substance ruptures, end-to-end sutures are used, while for ruptures closed to the osteotendinous junction, patellar drill holes or anchors are largely employed. Augmentation techniques are applied in presence of poor quality of tendon tissue or in case of delayed surgery, whenever a quadriceps retraction is present. Technical evolution of surgical materials has enabled an improvement in terms of results and biocompatibility [66–71].

After surgery, according to the biological processes of tendon healing and some clinical evidences, 6 weeks seems to be the most appropriate period of immobilization; after this period, it is essential to plan a proper and customized rehabilitative pathway for functional recovery of the knee, in order to prevent and/or avoid joint stiffness and functional impairment [23–28, 30].

References

1. La S, Fessell DP, Femino JE, Jacobson JA, Jamadar D, Hayes C (2003) Sonography of partial-thickness quadriceps tendon tears with surgical correlation. J Ultrasound Med 22(12):1323–1329; quiz 1330–1331
2. Tuong B, White J, Louis L, Cairns R, Andrews G, Forster BB (2011) Get a kick out of this: the spectrum of knee extensor mechanism injuries. Br J Sports Med 45(2):140–146. doi:10.1136/bjsm.2010.076695
3. Abram SG, Sharma AD, Arvind C (2012) Atraumatic quadriceps tendon tear associated with calcific tendonitis. BMJ Case Rep pii:bcr2012007031. doi:10.1136/bcr-2012-007031
4. Brukner P, Khan K (2012) Clinical sports medicine. 4th edn. McGraw-Hill Education, Australia
5. Kumar S, Rachakatla N, Kerin C, Kumar R (2010) Simultaneous traumatic rupture of the patellar tendon and the contralateral quadriceps tendon in a healthy individual. BMJ Case Rep pii:bcr0620103057. doi:10.1136/bcr.06.2010.3057
6. Hardy JR, Chimutengwende-Gordon M, Bakar I (2005) Rupture of the quadriceps tendon: an association with a patellar spur. J Bone Joint Surg Br 87(10):1361–1363
7. Clayton RA (2008) Court-Brown CM The epidemiology of musculoskeletal tendinous and ligamentous injuries. Injury 39(12):1338–1344. doi:10.1016/j.injury.2008.06.021
8. Maffulli N, Del Buono A, Spiezia F, Longo UG, Denaro V (2012) Light microscopic histology of quadriceps tendon ruptures. Int Orthop 36(11):2367–2371. doi:10.1007/s00264-012-1637-z
9. Ilan DI, Tejwani N, Keschner M, Leibman M (2003) Quadriceps tendon rupture. J Am Acad Orthop Surg 11(3):192–200
10. Ni Fhoghlu C, Ellanti P, Moriarity A, McCarthy T (2015) MRI features of a quadriceps tendon rupture. BMJ Case Rep pii:bcr2015209942. doi:10.1136/bcr-2015-209942
11. Longo UG, Fazio V, Poeta ML, Rabitti C, Franceschi F, Maffulli N, Denaro V (2009) Bilateral consecutive rupture of the quadriceps tendon in a man with BstUI polymorphism of the COL5A1 gene. Knee Surg Sports Traumatol Arthrosc 19(8):1403
12. Jolles BM, Garofalo R, Gillain L, Schizas C (2007) A new clinical test in diagnosing quadriceps tendon rupture. Ann R Coll Surg Engl 89(3):259–261
13. Arumilli B, Adeyemo F, Samarji R (2009) Bilateral simultaneous complete quadriceps rupture following chronic symptomatic tendinopathy: a case report. J Med Case Rep 3:9031. doi:10.4076/1752-1947-3-9031
14. Pfirrmann CW, Jost B, Pirkl C, Aitzetmüller G, Lajtai G (2008) Quadriceps tendinosis and patellar tendinosis in professional beach volleyball players: sonographic findings in correlation with clinical symptoms. Eur Radiol 18(8):1703–1709. doi:10.1007/s00330-008-0926-9
15. Sernik RA, Cerri GG (2010) Ultrasonografia del sistema muscoloscheletrico. *Correlazione con la risonanza magnetica*. Casa Editrice Piccin, Luglio
16. Kamel M, Eid H, Mansour R (2004) Ultrasound detection of knee patellar enthesitis: a comparison with magnetic resonance imaging. Ann Rheum Dis 63(2):213–214
17. Visnes H, Tegnander A, Bahr R (2015) Ultrasound characteristics of the patellar and quadriceps tendons among young elite athletes. Scand J Med Sci Sports 25(2):205–215. doi:10.1111/sms.12191

18. Kadakia NR, Ilahi OA (2003) Interobserver variability of the Insall-Salvati ratio. Orthopedics 26(3):321–323; discussion 323–324
19. Foley R, Fessell D, Yablon C, Nadig J, Brandon C, Jacobson J (2015) Sonography of traumatic quadriceps tendon tears with surgical correlation. J Ultrasound Med 34(5):805–810. doi:10.7863/ultra.34.5.805
20. Yu JS, Petersilge C, Sartoris DJ, Pathria MN, Resnick D (1994) MR imaging of injuries of the extensor mechanism of the knee. Radiographics 14(3):541–551
21. Bianchi S, Zwass A, Abdelwahab IF, Banderali A (1994) Diagnosis of tears of the quadriceps tendon of the knee: value of sonography. AJR Am J Roentgenol 162(5):1137–1140
22. Swamy GN, Nanjayan SK, Yallappa S, Bishnoi A, Pickering SA (2012) Is ultrasound diagnosis reliable in acute extensor tendon injuries of the knee? Acta Orthop Belg 78(6):764–770
23. Kountouris A, Cook J (2007) Rehabilitation of Achilles and patellar tendinopathies. Best Pract Res Clin Rheumatol 21(2):295–316
24. Pedrelli A, Stecco C, Day JA (2009) Treating patellar tendinopathy with Fascial Manipulation. J Bodyw Mov Ther 13(1):73–80. doi:10.1016/j.jbmt.2008.06.002
25. Kaux JF, Forthomme B, Namurois MH et al (2014) Description of a standardized rehabilitation program based on sub-maximal eccentric following a platelet-rich plasma infiltration for jumper's knee. Muscles Ligaments Tendons J 4(1):85–89. eCollection 2014
26. Dimitrios S, Pantelis M, Kalliopi S (2012) Comparing the effects of eccentric training with eccentric training and static stretching exercises in the treatment of patellar tendinopathy. A controlled clinical trial. Clin Rehabil 26(5):423–430. doi:10.1177/0269215511411114
27. Visnes H, Hoksrud A, Cook J, Bahr R (2005) No effect of eccentric training on jumper's knee in volleyball players during the competitive season: a randomized clinical trial. Clin J Sport Med 15(4):227–234
28. Rio E, Kidgell D, Purdam C et al (2015) Isometric exercise induces analgesia and reduces inhibition in patellar tendinopathy. Br J Sports Med 49(19):1277–1283. doi:10.1136/bjsports-2014-094386
29. Matava MJ (1996) Patellar tendon ruptures. J Am Acad Orthop Surg 4(6):287–296
30. Kubo K (2015) Effects of repeated concentric and eccentric contractions on tendon blood circulation. Int J Sports Med 36(6):481–484. doi:10.1055/s-0034-1398649
31. Enwemeka CS (1992) Functional loading augments the initial tensile strength and energy absorption capacity of regenerating rabbit Achilles tendons. Am J Phys Med Rehabil 71:31–38
32. Murrel GA, Lilly EG 3rd, Goldner RD, Seaber AV, Best TM (1994) Effects of immobilization on Achilles tendon healing in a rat model. J Orthop Res 12:582–591
33. Palmes D, Spiegel HU, Schneider TO, Langer M, Stratmann U, Budny T, Probst A (2002) Achilles tendon healing: long-term biomechanical effects of postoperative mobilization in a new mouse model. J Orthop Res 20:939–946
34. Eliasson P, Fahlgren A, Pasternak B, Aspenberg P (2007) Unloaded rat Achilles tendon continue to grow, but lose viscoelasticity. J Appl Physiol 103:459–463
35. Andersson T, Eliasson P, Aspenberg P (2009) Tissue memory in healing tendons: short loading episodes stimulate healing. J Appl Physiol 107:417–421
36. Molloy T, Wang Y, Murrell GAC (2003) The roles of growth factors in tendon and ligament healing. Sports Med 33(5):381–394
37. Aspenberg P (2007) Stimulation of tendon repair: mechanical loading, GDFs and platelets. A mini-review. Int Orthop (SICOT) 31:783–789
38. Lanzetti RM, Vadalà A, Morelli F et al (2013) Bilateral quadriceps rupture: results with and without Platelet-rich plasma. Healio Orthopedics 36(11):e1474–e1478
39. Loppini M, Maffulli N (2012) Conservative management of tendinopathy: an evidence-based approach. Muscles Ligaments Tendons J 1(4):134–137
40. Adelmario Cavalcanti Nogueira Junior and Manoel de Jesus Moura Junior (2015) The effects of laser treatment in tendinopathy: a systematic review. Acta Ortop Bras 23(1):47–49

41. Wang CJ (2012) Extracorporeal shockwave therapy in musculoskeletal disorders. J Orthop Surg Res 7:11
42. Notarnicola A, Moretti B (2012) The biological effects of ESWT on tendon tissue muscles. Ligaments and Tendons J 2(1):33–37
43. d'Agostino MC, Craig K, Tibalt E, Respizzi S (2015) Shock wave as biological therapeutic tool: From mechanical stimulation to recovery and healing, through mechanotransduction. Int J Surg 24(Pt B):147–153. doi:10.1016/j.ijsu.2015.11.030
44. Speed C (2014) A systematic review of shockwave therapies in soft tissue conditions: focusing on the evidence. Br J Sports Med 48(21):1538–1542
45. Haupt G (1997) Shock waves in orthopedics. Article in German. Urologe A 36(3):233–238
46. Mani-Babu S, Morrissey D, Waugh C, Screen H, Barton C (2015) The effectiveness of extracorporeal shock wave therapy in lower limb tendinopathy: a systematic review. Am J Sports Med 43(3):752–761
47. Chen YJ, Wang CJ, Yang KD, Kuo YR, Huang HC, Huang YT, Sun YC, Wang FS (2004) Extracorporeal shock waves promote healing of collagenase-induced Achilles tendinitis and increase TGF-beta1 and IGF-I expression. J Orthop Res 22(4):854–861
48. Han SH, Lee JW, Guyton GP, Parks BG, Courneya JP, Schon LC (2009) Effect of extracorporeal shock wave therapy on cultured tenocytes. "J. Leonard Goldner Award 2008". Foot Ankle Int 30(2):93–98
49. de Girolamo L, Stanco D, Galliera E, Viganò M, Lovati AB, Marazzi MG, Romeo P, Sansone V (2014) Soft-focused extracorporeal shock waves increase the expression of tendon-specific markers and the release of anti-inflammatory cytokines in an adherent culture model of primary human tendon cells. Ultrasound Med Biol 40(6):1204–1215
50. Vetrano M, d'Alessandro F, Torrisi MR, Ferretti A, Vulpiani MC, Visco V (2011) Extracorporeal shock wave therapy promotes cell proliferation and collagen synthesis of primary cultured human tenocytes. Knee Surg Sports Traumatol Arthrosc 19(12):2159–2168
51. Chao YH, Tsuang YH, Sun JS, Chen LT, Chiang YF, Wang CC, Chen MH (2008) Effects of shock waves on tenocyte proliferation and extracellular matrix metabolism. Ultrasound Med Biol 34(5):841–852
52. Leone L, Vetrano M, Ranieri D, Raffa S, Vulpiani MC, Ferretti A, Torrisi MR, Visco V (2012) Extracorporeal Shock Wave Treatment (ESWT) improves in vitro functional activities of ruptured human tendon-derived tenocytes. PLoS One 7(11), e49759
53. Zhang D, Kearney CJ, Cheriyan T, Schmid TM, Spector M (2011) Extracorporeal shockwave-induced expression of lubricin in tendons and septa. Cell Tissue Res 346(2):255–262. doi:10.1007/s00441-011-1258-7
54. Waugh CM, Morrissey D, Jones E, Riley GP, Langberg H, Screen HR (2015) In vivo biological response to extracorporeal shockwave therapy in human tendinopathy. Eur Cell Mater 29:268–280; discussion 280
55. Ibounig T, Simons TA (2015) Etiology, diagnosis and treatment of tendinous knee extensor mechanism injuries. Review article. Scand J Surg pii:1457496915598761
56. Ciriello V, Gudipati S, Tosounidis T et al (2012) Clinical outcomes after repair of quadriceps tendon rupture: a systematic review. Injury, Int J Care Injured 43:1931–1938
57. Wenzl ME, Kirchner R, Seide K et al (2004) Quadriceps tendon ruptures-is there a complete functional restitution? Injury, Int J Care Injured 35:922–926
58. Kelly DW, Carter VS, Jobe FW, Kerlan RK (1984) Patellar and quadriceps tendon ruptures:jumper's knee. Am J Sports Med 12(5):375–380
59. Yepes H, Tang M, Morris SF, Stanish WD (2008) Relationship between hypovascular zones and patterns of ruptures of the quadriceps tendon. J Bone Joint Surg 90:2135–2141
60. Ramseier LE, Werner CML, Heinzelmann M (2006) Quadriceps and patellar tendon rupture. Injury Int J Care Injured 37:516–519
61. Malta LMA, Gameiro VS, Sampaio EA et al (2014) Quadriceps tendon rupture in maintenance haemodialysis patients: Results of surgical treatment and analysis of risk factors. Injury, Int Care Injured 45:1970–1973

62. Ellanti P, Moriarity A, Wainberg N et al (2015) Association between patella spurs and quadriceps tendon ruptures. Muscles Ligaments and Tendons J 5(2):88–91
63. Boublik M, Schlegel TF, Koonce RC et al (2013) Quadriceps tendon injuries in National Football League Players. Am J Sports Med 41:1841
64. O'Shea K, Kenny P, Donovan J et al (2002) Outcomes following quadriceps tendon ruptures. Injury, Int Care Injured 33:257–260
65. Verdano MA, Zanelli M, Corsini T et al (2014) Quadriceps tendon tear rupture in healthy patients treated with patellar drilling holes: clinical and ultrasonographic analysis after 36 month of follow up. Muscles Ligaments and Tendons J 4(2):194–200
66. Maniscalco P, Bertone C, Rivera F, Bocchi L (2000) A new method of repair for quadriceps tendon ruptures. A case report. Panminerva Med 42:223–225
67. Kim TWB, Kamath AF, Israelite CL (2011) Suture anchor repair of quadriceps tendon rupture after total knee arthroplasty. J Arthroplasty 26(5):817–820
68. Richards DP, Barber FA (2002) Repair of quadriceps tendon ruptures using suture anchors. Arthroscopy 18(5):556–559
69. Petri M, Dratzidis A, Brand S et al (2015) Suture anchor repair yields better biomechanical properties than transosseous sutures in ruptured quadriceps tendons. Knee Surg Sports Traumatol Arthrosc 23:1039–1045
70. Lee D, Stinner D, Mir H (2013) Quadriceps and patellar tendon ruptures. J Knee Surg 26(5):301–308. doi:10.1055/s-0033-1353989
71. Hidetomo S, Yoichi S, Toshiaki Y, Shin Y, Takahiro S, Koji N, Hiroaki K, Kimio S (2015) Arthroscopic quadriceps tendon repair: two case reports. Case Rep Orthop 937581. Published online 2015 February 28. doi:10.1155/2015/937581
72. Volk WR, Yagnik GP, Uribe JW (2014) Complications in brief: quadriceps and patellar tendon tears. Clin Orthop Relat Res 472(3):1050–1057. doi:10.1007/s11999-013-3396-6
73. Ribbans WJ, Angus PD (1989) Simultaneous bilateral rupture of the quadriceps tendon. Br J Clin Pract 43:122–125
74. Shah MK (2002) Simultaneous bilateral rupture of quadriceps tendons: analysis of risk factors and associations. South Med J 95:860–866
75. Mosler E, Folkhard W, Knorzer E, Nemetschek-GanslerH NT, Koch MH (1985) Stress-induced molecular rearrangement in tendon collagen. J Mol Biol 182:589–596
76. Boudissa M, Roudet A, Rubens-Duval B, Chaussard C, Saragaglia D (2014) Acute quadriceps tendon ruptures: a series of 50 knees with an average follow-up of more than 6 years. Orthop Traumatol Surg Res 100(2):213–216

Chapter 7
Iliotibial Band Syndrome (ITBS)

Marco Merlo and Sergio Migliorini

Abstract Iliotibial band syndrome (ITBS) is an overuse injury caused by ripetitive friction of the iliotibial band and underlying bursa or lateral synovial recess across the lateral femoral epicondyle. ITBS is a well known cause of lateral knee pain in endurance sports and particularly in long distance runners. Friction occurs near foot strike, predominantly in the foot contact phase at, or slightly below, 30° of knee flexion. The development of ITBS is usually caused by a combination of intrinsic and extrinsic factors, and it must be evaluated also the biomechanics of running and the training program. Imaging (MRI, sonography) is not usually required to confirm the diagnosis of ITBS. The conservative treatment includes activity modification, soft tissue therapy, electrotherapeutic modalities, corticosteroid injection and correction of the biomechanical abnormalities. The personal ITB surgical release, performed by the authors, may be indicated if the conservative management fails and it is a safe procedure to return to practice sports at the same level.

7.1 Introduction

Iliotibial band syndrome (ITBS) is an overuse injury caused by repetitive friction of the iliotibial band (ITB) and underlying bursa across the lateral femoral epicondyle. ITBS is the most common causes of lateral knee pain in runners, with 12 %

M. Merlo (✉)
Department of Orthopaedics, Busto Arsizio General Hospital, Busto Arsizio, VA 21052, Italy
e-mail: dottormarcomerlo@gmail.com, marco.merlo@asst-valleolona.it

S. Migliorini
ITU International Triathlon Union, Maison du Sport, Av. de Rhodanie 54, Lausanne, Switzerland
e-mail: sermigliorini@alice.it

G.N. Bisciotti, P. Volpi (eds.), *The Lower Limb Tendinopathies*, Sports and Traumatology, DOI 10.1007/978-3-319-33234-5_7

incidence of all the overuse injuries related to running [1, 2]. Renne, in 1975, first described the ITBS in marines, who underwent to heavy endurance training [3]. Considering the success of road endurance races in these years, the ITBS diagnosis is now really frequent. Other sports disciplines are involved in that pathology, such as triathlon, football, and cycling.

7.2 Etiopathogenesis

The ITB is considered a continuation of the tendinous portion of the tensor fascia latae muscle and is indirectly attached to parts of the gluteus medius, gluteus maximus, and the vastus lateralis muscles. The intermuscular septum connects the ITB to the linea aspera femoris until just proximal to the femoral lateral epicondyle. Distally, the ITB spans out and inserts on the lateral border of the patella, the lateral patellar retinaculum, and Gerdy tibial tubercle. The ITB is only free from bony attachment between the superior aspect on the lateral femoral epicondyle and Gerdy tubercle [4, 5]. A bursa, like synovial tissue, insinuates under the ITB and acts as an interface between ITB and lateral femoral epicondyle [6].

The ITB assists the tensor fascia latae as it abducts the thigh and controls and decelerates adduction of the thigh.

With knee in full extension and until 20–30° flexion, the ITB lies anteriorly to the femoral lateral epicondyle and acts as an active knee extensor. From 20° to 30° of knee flexion, the ITB is posterior to the femoral lateral epicondyle and acts like an active knee flexor [7]. During walking and running, the ITB is an important stabilizer of the lower limb.

A biomechanical study of runners found that the posterior edge of the band impinges against the lateral epicondyle just after footstrike in the gait cycle, and the friction occurs at or at slightly less than 30° of knee flexion. Orchard [8] suggests that the impingement, in runners who had ITBS, occurs in the foot contact phase at an average $21.4° \pm 4.3°$ angle knee flexion, at or slightly below the 30° of flexion traditionally described in the literature (Fig. 7.1).

As in the other overuse injuries, the ITBS has intrinsic and extrinsic causes [9] (Table 7.1).

The most important extrinsic factors are the training errors (sudden increases in mileage or intensity, hill running and time trial training, lack of warm-up, insufficient muscle stretching execution, and bad shoes) inadequate to the running biomechanics. In a triathlon, the transition from cycling to running, with the change from concentric muscular contractions of cycling to eccentric contraction of running, and from unloaded cycling phase to the load state of running is an extremely delicate phase in which some kilometers are required to regain neuromuscular efficiency and elasticity indispensable for proper running style [10]. In this phase the inability to dissipate the load forces of the locomotor apparatus by the lower limb can favor the transmission of stress to the knee. The runner's training at lower pace and the high impact running style induce the friction of ITB with less than 30° knee flexion at the footstrike.

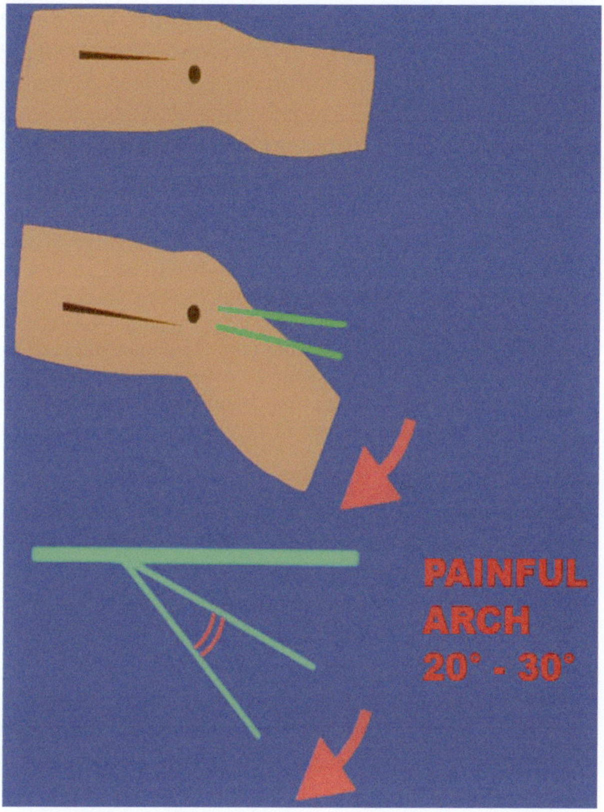

Fig. 7.1 During running the friction between ITB and lateral femoral epicondyle occurs at 20–30° of knee flexion

Table 7.1 ITBS intrinsic and extrinsic factors

Intrinsic	Extrinsic
Varus knee	High impact running styles
Internal tibial rotation	Training errors
Cavus-varus foot	Hill running
Femoral antetorsion	Insufficient muscle stretching
Knee lateral laxity	Bad or inadequate running shoes
Excessive foot pronation	Incorrect cleat pedal and saddle alignment
Hip abductors weakness	Cycling to running transition in triathlon
Lower leg discrepancies	

In cycling the abnormal lateral knee stress is most often the result of incorrect cleat pedal alignments, particularly with varus knee or external tibial rotation greater than 20°, when riding with internally rotated cleats. Generally this injury has increased since the introduction of rigid clip less pedal systems in 1985. Also a too high saddle results in the knee extension behind 150° causing the distal ITB to abrade across the lateral femoral epicondyle.

The surfaces of activity can also contribute to the development of ITBS in runners: running on surfaces with excessive camber can put excess strain on the lateral aspect of the knee. Downhill running tends to be worse because of the decrease in knee flexion that is present at the time of footstrike, thus increasing the force experienced by the knee within the Orchard impingement zone [8].

Anatomic factors that contribute to ITBS include excessive varus knee, excessive internal tibial torsion, foot pronation, hip abductor weakness, lower leg length discrepancies, cavus foot, femoral antetorsion. Fredericson [11] found that runners with ITBS had significant weakness in the hip abductors of their affected limb; the fatigued runner or those who have a weak gluteus medius are prone to increase thigh adduction and internal rotation at midstance, leading to an increased valgus vector at the knee. These condition increases tension on the ITB, making it more prone to impingement to the lateral femoral epicondyle, especially during the foot contact, when maximal deceleration absorbs ground reaction forces. In leg length discrepancy, the ITBS is more frequent in the lower leg due to the increasing of varus forefoot and increased knee Q angle [12].

Sixty five percent of athletes with ITBS are male, due to greater training volume and more number of practitioners [1]. In women the incidence of ITBS is less frequent than men because of anatomical factors: valgus knee, medial knee laxity, femoral lateral epicondyle less prominent.

Also the lack of muscular elasticity of the tensor fascia latae, knee, and hip flexors is an injury risk factor, particularly in the triathletes that compete in a triathlon after years of cycling competitions [10].

Other authors sustain a different pathogenesis of ITBS. Fairclough [13] suggests that ITB overuse injuries may be more likely to be associated with fat compression beneath the ITB rather than with repetitive friction as the knee flexes and extends. Ekman [14] and Hariri [15] consider that the inflammation of the bursa underlying the ITB is the only cause of ITBS.

7.3 Patient Evaluation

The main symptom of the ITBS is sharp pain or burning on the lateral aspect of the knee. The patient typically localizes the pain to the region of the distal ITB between the lateral femoral condyle and its insertion on the Gerdy tubercle. Runners often note that they start running pain-free but develop symptoms after a reproducible time or distance. If ITBS progresses, pain can persist even during walking, particularly when the patients ascent or descent stairs. In some cases the runner with ITBS can perform painless other sports activities, like skiing, basketball, and football.

The knee examination is typically negative except for local tenderness and, occasionally, swelling over the distal ITB where the band moves over the lateral femoral epicondyle.

Some provocative tests are commonly used in the assessment of ITBS and ITB function. Application of the direct pressure to the distal fibers across the lateral femoral epicondyle as the athletes flexed and extended the knee from 90° to 180° usually

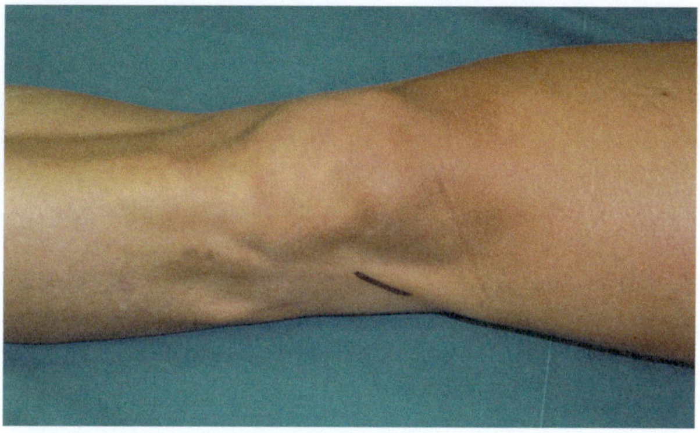

Fig. 7.2 Migliorini-Merlo sign. With the fully extended knee, it can observe an evident sulcus between the ITB and the lateral femoral epicondyle

elicited a very positive response (Holmes test). The Noble's test is performed with the patient lying supine; beginning with the affected knee flexed at 90°, the leg is extended with direct pressure over the lateral femoral epicondyle, with reproducible pain near 30° of knee flexion. The Thomas test is used to determine the tightness of the iliopsoas muscle, rectus femoris muscle, and ITB. The patient is instructed to lie supine at the edge of the examination table with both knees held to the chest. The patient holds the unaffected leg to the chest, and the affected leg is extended and lowered. A positive test results if the patient cannot completely extend and lower the affected leg to horizontal. Useful is also the Migliorini-Merlo sign: with the patient lying supine and the completely extended knee, it can be observed in the case of ITBS an evident sulcus between the ITB and the lateral femoral epicondyle (Fig. 7.2).

In particular cases it's important to perform an evaluation of biomechanics of running, evaluation of triathletes and cyclists on their bicycles, bikes, running shoes, orthosis, and shock absorbers review.

The differential diagnosis includes: lateral meniscal pathology, popliteal or biceps femoris tendinopathy, patellar syndrome, common peroneal nerve injury, lateral myofascial thigh pain, and osteochondral lesion of lateral femoral condyle.

7.4 Imaging

Although not routinely required, radiography imaging can be used to supplement the physical examination. Routine radiographs of the knee, including AP, lateral, and sunrise view can be used as a diagnostic adjunct to rule out other possible causes of the lateral knee pain, such as lateral joint space narrowing from degenerative disease, patellar maltracking, and stress fractures.

Ultrasonography of the knee lateral compartment is the first radiological evaluation considering low cost and availability of this modality compared with MRI. Usually ultrasonography performs a study to measure ITB thickness and the underlying bursa.

All athletes were examined with MRI to confirm the diagnosis because ITBS may be confused with other derangement of the knee, such as lateral meniscal tear, popliteal tendinopathy, lateral collateral ligament strain, hamstring strain, lateral femoral condyle osteochondral lesion, or transchondral fracture. Some authors [14, 16] reported the presence of high intensity signal, representing a fluid-filled collection, over the lateral epicondyle deep to the ITB as well as a marked thickening of the distal ITB. Eckman [14] demonstrated a significantly thicker ITB over the lateral femoral epicondyle. Thickness of the ITB in the disease group was 5.49±2.12 mm, as opposed to 2.52±1.56 mm in the control group.

7.5 Conservative Treatment

Nonsurgical management is the main stay of treatment of symptomatic ITBS.

In the acute phase the therapy must reduce the pain, and we suggest to rest from the inciting activities, such as running or cycling, for 2–3 weeks, until pain has resolved. Swimming with a pool buoy, without using lower extremities, normally is the only sport activity allowed in acute phase. Daily cryotherapy is useful in this phase and should be incorporated into the physical therapy program in an effort to reduce the inflammatory component of the ITBS.

Oral nonsteroidal anti-inflammatory drugs (NSAIDs) can be used to reduce the acute inflammatory response, and these alone have not been found to be effective in providing symptom relief. On the contrary local corticosteroid injections can relieve pain as well as aid in the diagnosis of ITBS, after 3 days of pain and, particularly, infiltrating the underlying bursa. Local corticosteroid infiltrations are effective and safe in the early (first 14 days) treatment of recent onset ITBS [17].

Therapy with platelet-rich plasma (PRP) should be an opportunity, but actually it needs more studies to determine the real efficacy.

Physical therapy is an important component of the nonsurgical management of ITBS. Typical regimens consist of specific stretching exercises focused on the ITB, tensor fascia latae, hamstrings, and gluteus medius. Stretching is indicated also for the iliopsoas, rectus femoris, and gastrocnemius and soleus muscles when restrictions are noted on physical examination. Stretching exercises are started after acute inflammation subsides. Additionally, the patient can use a foam roller as a myofascial release tool to break up soft-tissue adhesions in the ITB. In the subacute phase, it's important for the treatment of fascia lata and vastus lateralis trigger points with deep stripping massage, compression, fibrolysis, and mesotherapy. Shock waves should show good results if applied to the ITB and to the trigger points in the musculotendinous junction of the distal vastus lateralis. Manual therapy that consists of soft-tissue and medial patella mobilization may also contribute to lengthening the ITB.

Once the patient is capable of performing the stretching regimen without pain, strengthening is added to the rehabilitation program. Attention is paid to proximal strengthening of the hip abductors (gluteus medius) and the core muscles to stabilize the pelvis to prevent excessive adduction of the hip [7]. The initial exercise is side-lying leg lifts to help the patient learn to isolate the gluteus medius muscle. All strength exercises, should start with one set of 20 repetitions and build up to free sets of repetition daily. Because training is specific to limb position, it is essential that the patients progress to weight-bearing exercises. Initially the patients are asked to perform a step-down exercise; once this is mustered patients are taught to perform the pelvic drop exercises [11].

During the subacute phase, the athlete can return to cycling, easy pedaling (80 rpm or less) with a little resistance at a pain-free cadence on flat terrains. Return to running depends on the severity of the condition and patient's premorbid function. We recommend running, every 2 days, starting with easy sprints on level ground over slow jogging; biomechanical studies have shown that faster-paced running is less likely to aggravate the ITBS [8]. We suggest gradual increase in distance running and frequency, avoiding hill training and intensive training (too much, too soon). Most of the patients have symptomatic relief without surgery within 6–8 weeks and are capable of returning to their athletic activities with no long-term sequelae.

Great attention should be focused on sport equipment, considering running shoes and biomechanics of the foot contact on the ground, the bike saddle position (avoiding knee extension beyond 150°), and the incorrect cleat pedal alignment (varus knee or external tibial rotation more then 20 % causes a significant stress on distal ITB when riding with internally rotated cleats). The hyperpronated runner should use stable running shoes and change the shoes every 500–600 miles, considering that shoes lose almost 60 % of their capacity to absorb ground reaction forces [18].

Length discrepancies of the lower legs should be corrected with orthosis for the running shoes or with thickness between cycling shoes and cleat pedals. In some cases it is useful putting inside the shoes the shock absorbers, in order to increase the knee flexion at the footstrike.

7.6 Surgical Treatment

Surgical treatment is indicated only after extensive nonoperative measures have failed to relieve symptoms (3–6 months).

Holmes [19] suggests two procedures: percutaneous release and the open release excision. The percutaneous incision is performed under local anesthetic with the knee held at 90° so that the posterior fibers are free from the lateral femoral epicondyle. The open release surgery consists of the excision of an ellipse tissue measuring 4 cm at the base and 2 cm at the apex.

Martens [20] resected from the posterior part of the ITB a triangular portion 2-cm wide at the posterior base and 1.5-cm in height. The ITB Z-lengthening is also an option described by Richards [9]. Hariri [15] suggests an open ITB bursectomy. Michels [21] described an arthroscopic technique to treat refractory ITBS using a synovial shaver to resect the lateral synovial recess accessed through an accessory superolateral portal.

Our personal surgical procedure, usually in local anesthesia and in day surgery hospital, is performed by a small access (less than 2 cm) and consists of a subtotal vertical tenotomy of the ITB with the knee held at 70° of flexion. We don't remove the bursa underlying the ITB because of the high risk of hematoma and persistent synovial reaction. The ITB release is sufficient to remove the ITB impingement with the lateral femoral epicondyle and consequent reduction of the bursitis. Compression bandage and cryotherapy is mandatory at the end of the procedure. In some cases we perform an arthroscopic evaluation of the knee joint to rule out other associated articular lesions, particularly involving the lateral meniscus (Fig. 7.3).

Postoperative protocol began immediately after surgery. Patients are allowed to be weight-bearing as tolerated with bilateral crutches until their gait normalized. Typically they are able to walk without crutches between 3 and 5 days postoperatively. Some athletes develop small seromas or hematomas near the incision during the 2nd postoperative week. These resolved spontaneously in 3–5 days with intermittent icing, local compresses, or aspiration. Passive range of motion for the hip and knee began on postoperative day 1 with full knee extension achieved by day 3 and full hip and knee flexion by the end of week 2. Patellofemoral joint mobilizations are also performed with specific emphasis on medial glides of the patella. A gentle massage and range of motion for the ITB are initiated in week 1 and progressed to gradual stretching in week 2.

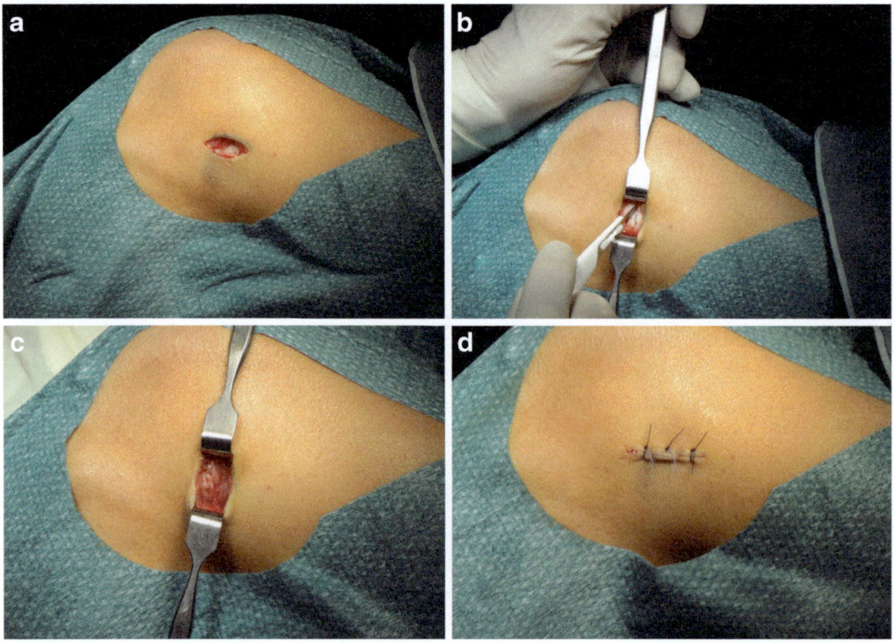

Fig. 7.3 Our personal procedure. (**a**) Approach to ITB; (**b**) vertical incision of ITB; (**c**) complete release of ITB; (**d**) skin suture

Isometric exercises for the hip abductors are performed during week 1 and progressed to active range of motion and progressive resisted isotonic exercises during week 2–4. The initial exercise is side-lying leg lifts to help the patient learn to isolate the gluteus medius muscle. For all strength exercises, the patients start with one set of 20 repetitions and build up to 3 sets of 20 repetitions daily. Because training is specific to limb position, it is essential that patients progress to weight-bearing exercises. Initially, athletes perform step-down exercises. Once this is mastered, patients are taught to perform the pelvic drop exercises. Neuromuscular electrical stimulation is applied to the quadriceps to prevent the effects of postoperative inhibition. The patients are revaluated by the operating surgeon at week 4 and cleared to begin a gradual progression of swimming and cycling as tolerated with a return to running between 6 and 8 weeks postoperatively. As a general rule, athletes can return to running once they can perform all strength exercises without pain. We recommend running every other day for the first 4 weeks, starting with easy sprints on level ground. Biomechanical studies [8] have shown that faster-paced running is less likely to aggravate ITBS because at footstrike the knee is flexed beyond the angles that cause friction. In our experience, according to Evans [4], the ITB release does not affect the biomechanics of the hip and knee.

7.7 Conclusions

ITBS is a common cause of lateral knee pain in the athletic patients' population, particularly in endurance sports. We focus the importance of the exact etiology underlying the condition that it is different for every athlete considering the intrinsic and extrinsic factors. Most patients with ITBS improve with aggressive protocol rehabilitation and activity modification. Surgery release of the ITB is indicated only after extensive nonoperative measures have failed to relieve symptoms. Between a variety of surgical management options, our personal surgical procedure reported good results and return athletes to pain-free athletic activity.

Bibliography

1. Barber FA, Sutker AN (1992) Iliotibial band syndrome. Sports Med 14(2):144–148
2. Noble CA (1980) Iliotibial band friction in runners. Am J Sports Med 8:232–234
3. Renne JW (1975) The iliotibial band friction syndrome. J Bone Joint Surg Am 57(8):1110–1111
4. Evans P (1979) The postural function, of the iliotibial tract. Ann R Coll Surg Engl 61(4):272–280
5. Terry GC, Hughston JC, Norwood LA (1986) The anatomy of the iliopatellar band and the iliotibial tract. Am J Sports Med 14(1):39–45
6. Nemeth WC, Sanders BL (1996) The lateral synovial recess of the knee: anatomy and role in chronic iliotibial band friction syndrome. Arthroscopy 12(5):574–580

7. Strauss EJ, Kim S, Calcei JC, Park D (2011) Iliotibial band syndrome: evaluation and management. J Am Acad Orthop Surg 19(12):728–736
8. Orchard JW, Fricker PA, Abud AT, Mason BR (1996) Biomechanics of iliotibial band friction syndrome in runners. Am J Sports Med 24(3):375–379
9. Orava S, Lappilahti J (1999) Overuse injuries of tendons in athletes. J Bone Joint Surg (Br) 4:128–131
10. Migliorini S (2000) The triathlon: acute and overuse injuries. J Sports Traumatol Relat Res 22(4):186–195
11. Fredericson M, Guillet M, De Benedictis L (2000) Quick solutions for iliotibial band syndrome. Phys Sports Med 28(2):55–68
12. Schwellnus MP (1993) Lower limb biomechanics in runners with the iliotibial band friction syndrome. Med Sci Sports Exerc 25(5):S69
13. Fairclough JJ, Hayashi K, Toumi H, Lyons K, Bydder G, Phillips N, Best TM, Benjamin M (2006) The functional anatomy of the iliotibial band during flexion and extension of the knee: implications for understanding iliotibial band syndrome. J Anat 208(3):309–316
14. Ekman EF, Pope T, Martin DF, Curl WW (1994) Magnetic resonance imaging of the iliotibial band syndrome. Am J Sports Med 22:851–854
15. Hariri S, Savidge ET, Reinold MM, Zachazewski J, Gill TJ (2009) Treatment of recalcitrant iliotibial band friction syndrome with open iliotibial band bursectomy. Am J Sports Med 37(7):1417–1424
16. Murphy BJ, Hechtman KS, Uribe JW, Selesnick H, Smith RL, Zlatkin MB (1992) Iliotibial band friction syndrome: MR imaging findings. Radiology 185(2):569–571
17. Gunter P, Schwellnus MP (2004) Local corticosteroid injection in iliotibial band friction syndrome in runners: a randomised controlled trial. Br J Sports Med 38:269–272
18. Cook SD, Kester MA, Brunet ME, Haddad RJ Jr (1985) Biomechanics of running shoe performance. Clin Sports Med 4:619–626
19. Holmes JC, Pruitt AL, Whalen NJ (1993) Iliotibial band syndrome in cyclists. Am J Sports Med 21(3):419–424
20. Martens M, Libbrecht P, Burssens A (1989) Surgical treatment of iliotibial band friction syndrome. Am J Sports Med 17(5):651–654
21. Michels F, Jambon S, Allard M, Bousquet T, Colombet P, De Lavigne C (2009) An artroscopic technique to treat the ileotibial band syndrome. Knee Surg Sports Traumatol Arthrosc 17(3):233–236

Chapter 8
Hamstring Syndrome

Gian Nicola Bisciotti, L. Pulici, A. Quaglia, A. Orgiani, L. Balzarini, P. Felisaz, and Piero Volpi

Abstract The hamstring syndrome is classically considered an insertional tendinopathy concerning the proximal hamstrings. However, we must not forget its possible posttraumatic cause. In effect, its association with previous proximal hamstring lesion is well described in literature. It is a typical sport pathology that mainly affects sprinters, distance runners, soccer players, and nordic skiers. Its greatest incidence is between 29 and 37 years old. The first-choice treatment is conservative and the surgical treatment can be considered only in the case of a failure of conservative treatment.

8.1 Introduction

The hamstring syndrome (HS) was described for the first time from Puranen and Orawa in 1988 [1] and is considered an insertional tendinopathy of proximal hamstrings. Usually HS is associated to a previous proximal hamstring lesion with the production of fibrotic tissue or to a degenerative process that causes a widening of the proximal hamstring tendon which causes an irritation of the near sciatic nerve [1, 3]. The association with previous proximal hamstring lesion is well described [1, 3–7] and it represents from 19 to 76 % of cases [2, 5, 8–12]. At the beginning the HS

G.N. Bisciotti (✉)
Qatar Orthopaedic and Sports Medicine Hospital, FIFA Center of Excellence, Doha, Qatar
e-mail: bisciotti@libero.it

L. Pulici • A. Quaglia • A. Orgiani • L. Balzarini • P. Felisaz
Humanitas Clinical Institute, IRCCS, Rozzano, Milan, Italy

P. Volpi
Humanitas Clinical Institute, IRCCS, Rozzano, Milan, Italy

FC Internazionale Medical staff, Milan, Italy

G.N. Bisciotti, P. Volpi (eds.), *The Lower Limb Tendinopathies*,
Sports and Traumatology, DOI 10.1007/978-3-319-33234-5_8

was described as a sprinter's pathology [1], but our current knowledge is that this pathology is much frequent in distance runners, soccer players, and nordic skiers [1, 2, 5, 7]. The higher incidence is between 29 and 37 years old [5, 11, 13].

8.2 Clinical Diagnosis

Most patients with HS had an elective pain, with different intensity, when palpating proximal hamstring insertion [1, 2, 5, 7, 11], while manual tests of hamstrings or gluteal muscles can be normal [3, 8]. Also neurological tests are negative [5, 8]. Usually the patient refers a discomfort at proximal hamstring insertion during the test of flexibility, but these tests couldn't show a significant deficit [1, 5]. The hamstring-stretch test (HST) (Fig. 8.1) is positive if it evokes pain at proximal hamstring insertion [7]. Other similar tests are the Puranen-Orawa test (Fig. 8.2) and the bent-knee stretch test (Fig. 8.3). Since it often involves a hypotrophy of the abductor hip muscles [14], the Trendelenburg test could be positive at the affected site [2]. According to the involvement of sciatic nerve, patients can show a different grade

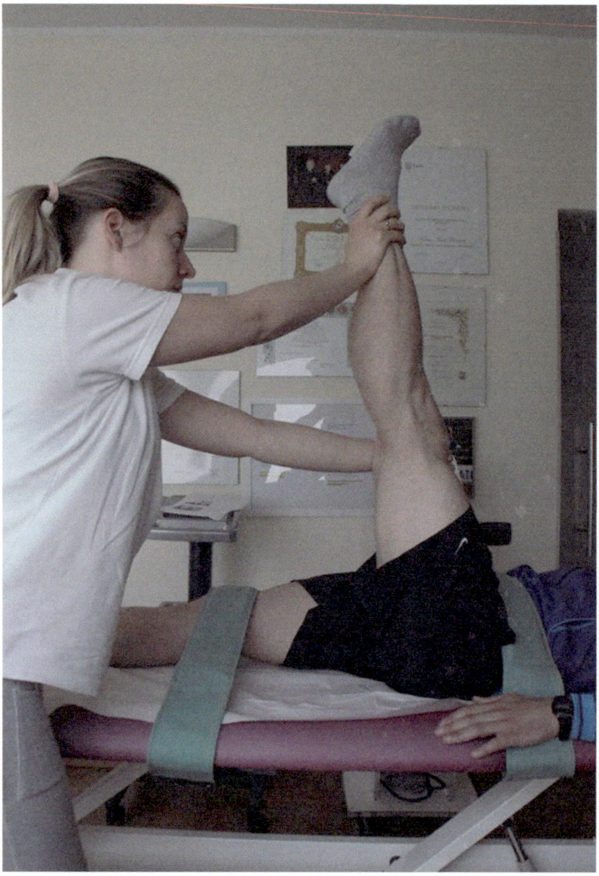

Fig. 8.1 In the hamstring-stretch test, the operator makes a rapid hip flexion followed immediately by an equally rapid extension of the knee. It is positive if it evokes pain at proximal hamstring insertion

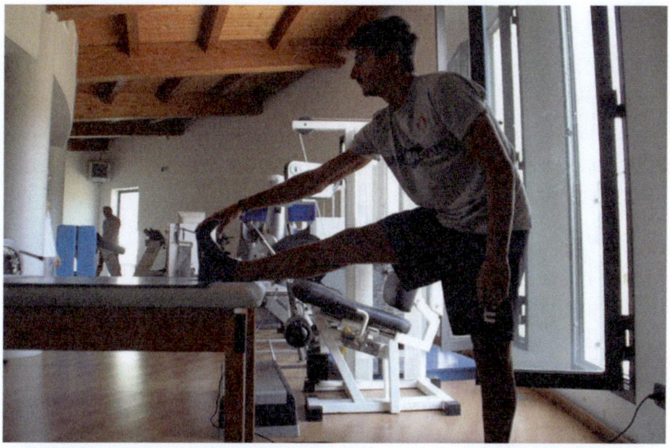

Fig. 8.2 In the Puranen-Orawa test, the patient makes an active stretching of hamstrings during stance. It is positive if it evokes pain at proximal hamstring insertion

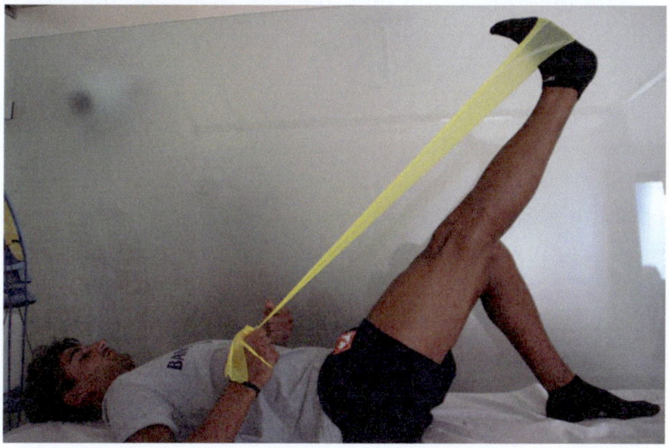

Fig. 8.3 In the bent-knee stretch test, the patient makes, using a band, a stretching of hamstring in supine position. It is positive if it evokes pain at proximal hamstring insertion

of radicular symptoms. Generally HS does not interfere with running but limits it greatly. Usually pain is evoked by running uphill and downhill and during sprinting, remaining "low" during running at low velocity and on flat ground. Other symptom referred is pain at ischiatic tuberosity when patients maintain sitting position especially on hard surfaces [2]. Differential diagnosis should consider [15]:

- Indirect lesions of hamstrings
- Piriform syndrome
- Ischiatic bursitis
- Sciatica
- Chronic compartment syndrome of the thigh
- Deep hematomas
- Soft tissue neoplasia

8.3 Imaging

Pathology of the hamstring complex may affect the cancellous bone and the cortex of the ischial tuberosity, the tendons, the myotendinous junction, the perimysial fascia, the muscle, and finally the sciatic nerve.

The diagnostic imaging approach requires high tissue contrast resolution, safety, and favorable cost/benefit ratio modalities.

Today MRI is considered the gold standard in diagnostic imaging.

Conventional plain films may play a role in detecting cortical bone changes and soft tissue calcifications adjacent to the ischial tuberosity, which are typical signs of chronic enthesopathy, typically seen in elderly patients. Conventional radiography allows also visualization of avulsed bone fragments in posttraumatic injuries.

CT should be limited to selected cases because of the poor soft tissue contrast and the high radiation dose on the pelvis. Nonetheless it may be required to better define the anatomy of an avulsed bone fragment.

Ultrasound is a safe technique, sensitive for the study of superficial structures such as the tendons, but do not provide information on the cancellous bone. Furthermore it suffers of inter-operator variability and hence skilled operators are required.

The imaging technique that can overview all such pathologic changes is MRI, with adequate detection of bone marrow edema, tendons or muscle strains or tears, and scar tissue formation.

MRI is a safe, repeatable examination with low inter-operator variability and allows great definition of the anatomy for the surgical repair.

On the coronal plane, the ischial tuberosity presents two facets; the superolateral or oblique facet is the side of attachment of the semimembranosus, while the inferomedial or horizontal facet is the side where the biceps femoris and the semitendinosus tendons attach as a conjoint tendon. Sometimes these two tendons are difficult to separate, reflecting anatomic variation. The tendon attachments are best seen in the coronal plane but verification of the findings in the axial plane is very important. The radiologist must be aware of the attachment of the adductor magnum tendon at the inferomedial facet, which is intimately associated with the conjoint tendon, just adjacent to it but slight medially and anteriorly located, which may be a source of misdiagnosis if confused.

The type of injury is most easily defined with MRI, which in most cases does not require contrast injection. Hamstring injuries may be classified in strains (or partial tears) and avulsion (or complete tears).

Most strains occur in the region of the myotendinous junction (MTJ) [16], which is the weakest area linked to the muscle. However, the MTJ is not a distinct area but a 10–12-cm zone of transition in which muscle fibrils intersect with the tendon origin or ligamentous insertion. Hyperintensity in T2 fat suppressed or STIR images is typical of edema, fluid, and blood products that are commonly displayed between intact muscle fibers, creating a feathered appearance. Hemorrhage may be more important with major muscle strain; it is typically hyperintense in the acute setting and may track around the sciatic nerve.

Hamstring avulsion is defined by the detachment of one or more proximal tendons of the hamstring from the flat bony surfaces of the ischial tuberosity. In adults complete avulsion usually involves the tendons but not the bone. Tendon avulsion must be recognized with specification of the degree of retraction because it necessitates prompt surgical repair. Complete avulsion almost always involves the conjoint tendon (biceps femoris and semitendinosus) and most frequently a partial avulsion of the semimembranosus. The avulsion of all the three tendons is also common, while avulsion at one or two attachments is less frequent [17].

Acute injuries in pediatric patients often result with a bone fragment avulsion, detectable on plain films and by US.

In the immature skeleton, the apophysis forms the weakest link in the musculo-tendinous unit due to its incomplete ossification; these injuries sometimes lead to a large bone formation because of the typical great vascularity of the avulsed ossification center [18]. It is important to determine whether the attachment side is displaced more than 2 cm [19].

Chronic tears of the hamstring complex can be investigated with MRI to evaluate scar tissue formation. This scar tissue has low signal intensity with all pulse sequences.

On MRI long-standing injuries lead to disuse changes such as atrophy of the muscles with fatty replacement, best demonstrated on T1-weighted MR images. The sciatic nerve should be routinely assessed to demonstrate potential encasement, compression, or tethering.

On US the scar tissue is characterized by irregular shape and heterogeneous echotexture. Diffuse and focal thickening with hypoechoic change is characteristic of chronic tendinopathy. US combines good spatial resolution, with the ability of dynamic assessment that may provide additional useful information about the tendon integrity. Fluid collections around the tendons may be easily demonstrated. Contralateral evaluation is useful for comparison.

MTJ tears can be subtle at MR imaging and even more at US, because of the low contrast between the muscle and the interfascicular edema. Nevertheless, US is a sensitive imaging modality in the presence of blood products and edema, which increase with the conspicuity of muscle disruption. Color Doppler US can be used to assess neovascularization, inflammation, and healing, while elastography may theoretically assess the degree of muscle edema or connective tissue substitution.

8.4 Conservative Treatment

Conservative treatment is the first approach for HS; it should consider these points:

- A pelvic alignment
- Soft tissue mobilization
- Active and passive stretching of hamstring muscles
- Eccentric training of hamstring muscles
- Core stability

The extracorporeal shock wave therapy has limited evidence even if a recent study [7] showed possible benefit. Local injection of corticosteroids has a positive outcome in little more than 20 %, and the symptomatic relief is not more than 6 months [13]. Regenerative therapy, based on platelet-rich plasma, nowadays didn't show sufficient scientific evidence [20].

The eccentric training of hamstring muscles is the focus of the rehabilitation program [21–26]. None of the authors cited suggest the elimination of concentric phase during the exercises proposed, but they underline the importance of improving the eccentric phase with a reduction of the concentric one. According to our experience, eccentric isokinetic exercises should be completed with isotonic exercises promoting eccentric phase.

We propose some exercises very helpful into the conservative treatment of HS (Figs. 8.4, 8.5, 8.6, and 8.7). This kind of exercise can be introduced as soon as the

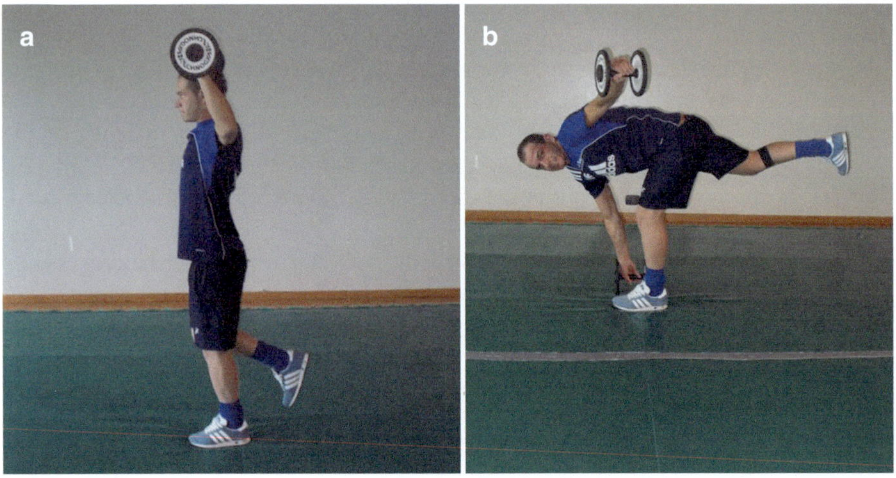

Fig. 8.4 Single-limb balance windmill touches with dumbbells: begin in (**a**) single-limb stance position with dumbbells overhead and (**b**) perform windmill motion under control with end position of touching dumbbell to the floor

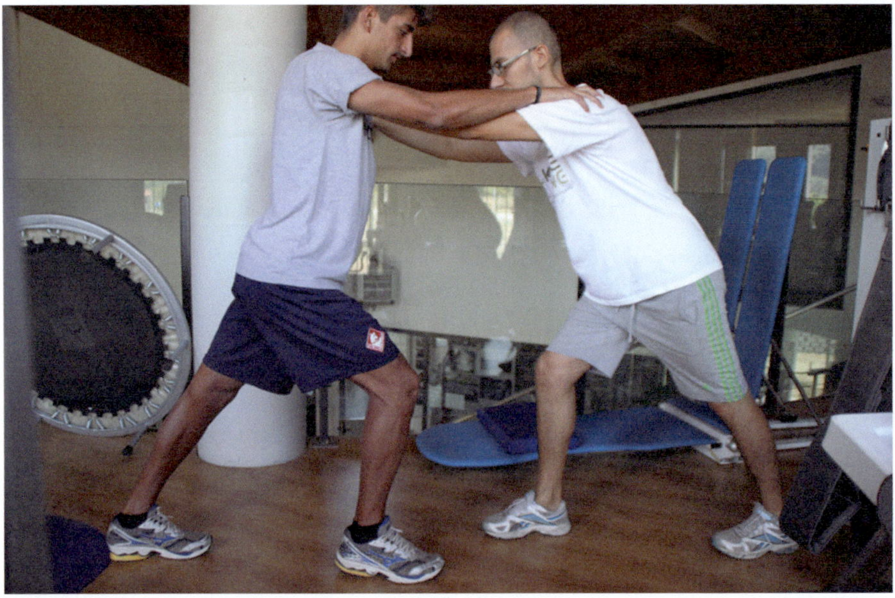

Fig. 8.5 Eccentric backward steps. The subject resists the clinician attempt to push him/her backward. The injured leg is held back

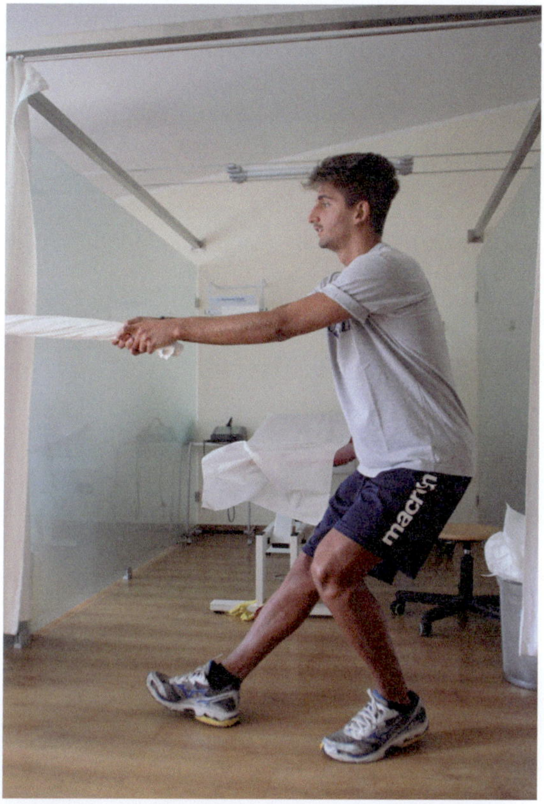

Fig. 8.6 Eccentric forward pulls. The subject resists forward pull by the clinician

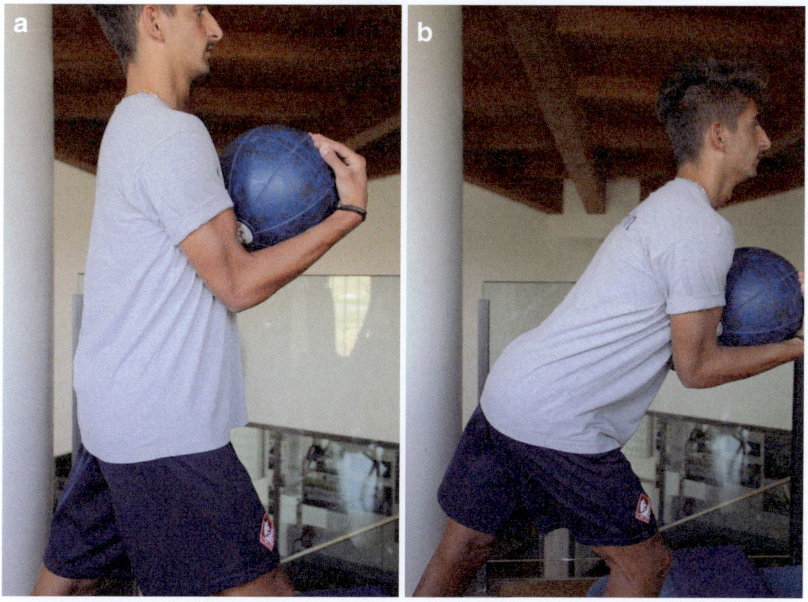

Fig. 8.7 Split stance exercise also called the "good morning" exercise. The subject is in a split stance position with the weight placed anteriorly to increase the lever arm on the hamstrings (**a**). The subject then leans forward through flexion at the hip (**b**)

first part of the conservative program, based on weight-bearing exercises made at low velocity, is tolerated from patients without discomfort [27].

Further the exercises described above, we find very interesting the introduction of a workout based on whole-body vibrations (WBV) (Figs. 8.8, 8.9, 8.10, 8.11, and 8.12). There are some studies that show how the WBV are able to improve elongation capacity of hamstrings [28, 29]. This effect is attributable to the myorelaxant effect induced by vibration at particular frequency (18–20 Hz) [30]. According to this aspect of WBV, we recommend the introduction of this program [31, 32] into the conservative treatment of HS.

8.5 Surgical Treatment

A surgical approach to HS is not often easy to choose. Obviously this choice is limited to those cases where the conservative treatment has failed [5, 11]. In the preoperative evaluation, the close proximity between the proximal insertion of hamstrings and the sciatic nerve should be taken into account, because an edematous or thickened tendon can compress the sciatic nerve or could form adhesion between these structures [5].

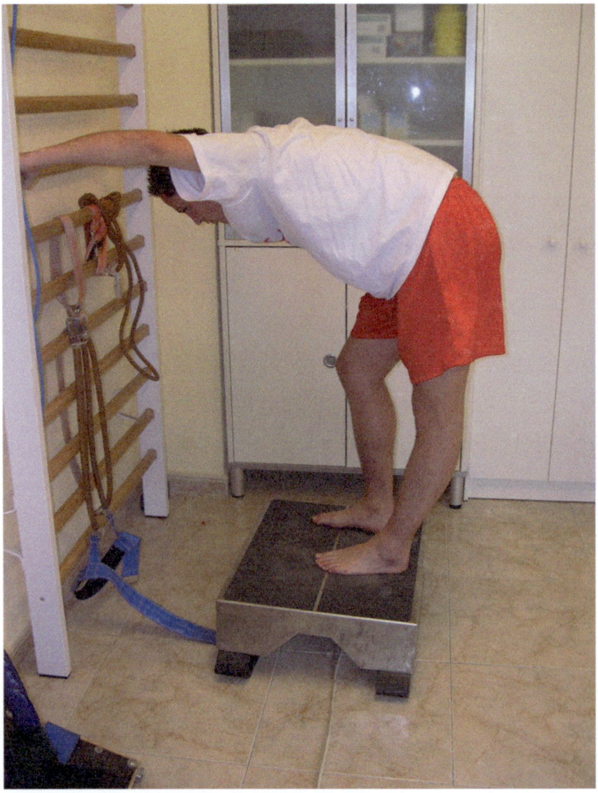

Fig. 8.8 Stretching of posterior kinetic chain. The subject must make a flexion/extension of the patella, forcing an extension to increase the stretch of the muscle tendon complex
Frequency, from 18 to 20 Hz
Vibration amplitude, from 2 to 3 mm
Acceleration peak, between 25.5 m.s–2 (2.6 g) and 47 m.s–2 (4.8 g)
Set, from 3 to 5
Working time, 1′
Rest time, 2′

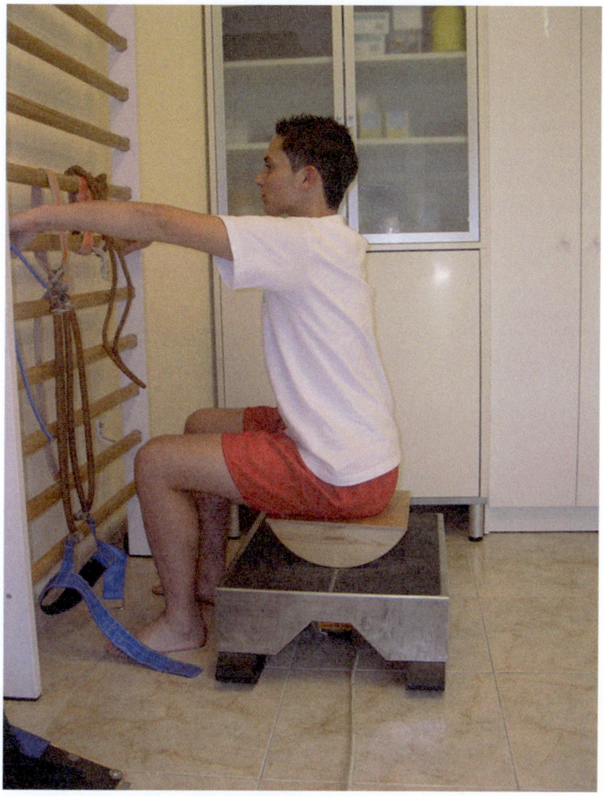

Fig. 8.9 Stretching of paravertebral muscle with Freeman platform, combined with vibrations. It's important to combine a full expiration to the muscular spine stretching
Frequency, from 18 to 20 Hz
Vibration amplitude, from 2 to 3 mm
Acceleration peak, between 25.5 m.s–2 (2.6 g) and 47 m.s–2 (4.8 g)
Set, from 3 to 5; working time, 1′
Rest time, 2′

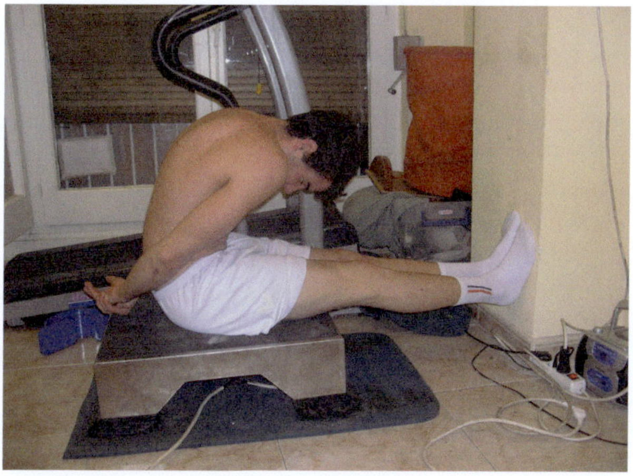

Fig. 8.10 Stretching exercise for back chain muscle
Frequency, from 18 to 20 Hz
Vibration amplitude, from 2 to 3 mm
Acceleration peak, between 25.5 m.s–2 (2.6 g) and 47 m.s–2 (4.8 g)
Set, from 3 to 5; working time, 1′
Rest time, 2′

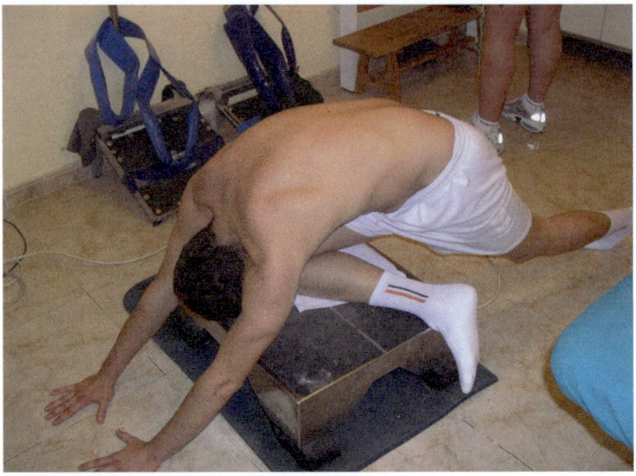

Fig. 8.11 Stretching exercise of piriformis muscle and sacrotuberous ligament
Frequency, from 18 to 20 Hz
Vibration amplitude, from 2 to 3 mm
Acceleration peak, between 25.5 m.s–2 (2.6 g) and 47 m.s–2 (4.8 g)
Set, from 3 to 5; working time, 1′
Rest time, 2′

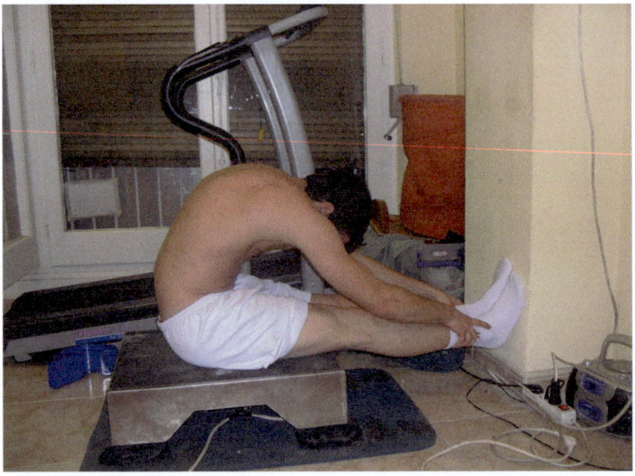

Fig. 8.12 Prolonged stretching exercise of posterior kinetic chain
Frequency, from 18 to 20 Hz
Vibration amplitude, from 2 to 3 mm
Acceleration peak, between 25.5 m.s–2 (2.6 g) and 47 m.s–2 (4.8 g); set, from 3 to 5
Working time, 1′
Rest time, 2′

The patient is positioned in the prone position. As surgical approach, a transverse incision along the gluteal fold or a posterior longitudinal approach can be used. To identify the proximal insertion of the hamstrings, the lower edge of the gluteus maximum should be moved proximally, after identification of the posterior femoral cutaneous nerve. At this point a transverse tenotomy of semimembranosus muscle at about 3–4 cm from its origin can be performed, and the biceps femoris and semitendinosus muscles were left intact. The tendon sectioned is fixed to biceps femoris to avoid excessive retraction. Once the tendon is sutured, the sciatic nerve is explored and it is released from any adhesions.

Postoperative treatment consists of an elastic bandage for about 2 weeks and a progressive load until reaching the full weight bearing in about 2 weeks. Swimming is allowed in 2 weeks from surgery while isometric exercises and cycling at 4 weeks. Running and more intensive workouts can be performed after 2 months. The return to sport is after at least 2 months.

The rehabilitation period after surgery lasts between 60 and 90 days, and the follow-up (2–10 years) report results defined as "excellent" or "good" between 77 and 88 % of the cases considered.

8.6 Conclusion

The HS diagnosis is not easy, and for this reason it can often be misunderstood. Often a HS framework is interpreted as a simple tendinopathy or an indirect muscle injury; as consequence the therapeutic process is based on a misdiagnosis. This leads to a lengthening of recovery times and especially to the risk of a disease chronicity. In this case a careful evaluation of the patient's medical history can help the clinician in identifying the correct diagnosis. Upon reaching a definitive diagnosis (that is possible only after the exclusion of all differential diagnoses), the patient must be routed, as first choice, to a conservative treatment. In any case the clinic and the patient should be aware that the conservative treatment involves a long and complex pathway. The surgical treatment is limited only when any type of conservative treatment is completely failed.

Note The authors thank Dr. Jose Manuel Sanchez (Centro de Alto Rendimiento de Barcelona) for the use of the Figs. 8.8, 8.9, 8.10, 8.11, and 8.12.

Bibliography

1. Puranen J, Orava S (1988) The hamstring syndrome. A new diagnosis of gluteal sciatic pain. Am J Sports Med 16(5):517–521
2. Fredericson M, Moore W, Guillet M, Beaulieu C (2005) High hamstring tendinopathy in runners: meeting the challenges of diagnosis, treatment, and rehabilitation. Phys Sportsmed 33(5):32–43
3. Sherry M (2012) Examination and treatment of hamstring related injuries. Sports Health 4(2):107–114
4. Askling CM, Tengvar M, Saartok T, Thorstensson A (2006) Acute first-time hamstring strains during high-speed running: a longitudinal study including clinical and magnetic resonance imaging findings. Am J Sports Med 35(2):197–206
5. Lempainen L, Sarimo J, Mattila K, Vaittinen S, Orava S (2009) Proximal hamstring tendinopathy: results of surgical management and histopathologic findings. Am J Sports Med 37(4):727–733
6. Saikku K, Vasenius J, Saar P (2010) Entrapment of the proximal sciatic nerve by the hamstring tendons. Acta Orthop Belg 76(3):321–324
7. Cacchio A, Rompe JD, Furia JP, Susi P, Santilli V, De Paulis F (2011) Shockwave therapy for the treatment of chronic proximal hamstring tendinopathy in professional athletes. Am J Sports Med 39(1):146–153
8. Agre JC (1985) Hamstring injuries. Proposed aetiological factors, prevention, and treatment. Sports Med 2(1):21–33
9. Hartig DE, Henderson JM (1999) Increasing hamstring flexibility decreases lower extremity overuse injuries in military basic trainees. Am J Sports Med 27(2):173–176

10. Clark RA (2008) Hamstring injuries: risk assessment and injury prevention. Ann Acad Med Singapore 37(4):341–346
11. Young IJ, van Riet RP, Bell SN (2008) Surgical release for proximal hamstring syndrome. Am J Sports Med 36(12):2372–2378
12. Benazzo F, Zanon MG, Indino C, Pelillo F (2013) Surgical management of chronic proximal hamstring tendinopathy in athletes: a 2 to 11 years of follow-up. J Orthopaed Traumatol 14:83–89
13. Zissen MH, Wallace G, Stevens KJ, Fredericson M, Beaulieu CF (2010) High hamstring tendinopathy: MRI and ultrasound imaging and therapeutic efficacy of percutaneous corticosteroid injection. AJR Am J Roentgenol 195(4):993–998
14. Patil S, Dixon J, White LC, Jones AP, Hui AC (2011) An electromyographic exploratory study comparing the difference in the onset of hamstring and quadriceps contraction in patients with anterior knee pain. Knee 18(5):329–332
15. Brandser E, El-Khoury G, Kathol M, Callaghan J, Tearse D (1995) Hamstring injuries: radiographic, conventional tomographic, CT, and MR imaging characteristics. Semin Musculoskel Radiol 197:257–262
16. Koulouris G, Connell D (2005) Hamstring muscle complex: an imaging review. Radiographics 25(3):571–586
17. Hong RJ, Hughes TH, Gentili A, Chung CB (2008) Magnetic resonance imaging of the hip. J Magn Reson Imaging 27(3):435–445
18. Chang GH, Paz DA, Dwek JR, Chung CB (2013) Lower extremity overuse injuries in pediatric athletes: clinical presentation, imaging findings, and treatment. Clin Imaging 37(5):836–846
19. Servant CT, Jones CB (1998) Displaced avulsion of the ischial apophysis: a hamstring injury requiring internal fixation. Br J Sports Med 32(3):255–257
20. Bisciotti GN (2013) I tendini. Biologia, patologia, aspetti clinici. Volume 1 (Anatomia ed aspetti generali). Calzetti e Mariucci Eds. Perugia
21. Askling C, Karlsson J, Thorstensson A (2003) Hamstring injury occurrence in elite soccer players after preseason strength training with eccentric overload. Scand J Med Sci Sports 13:244–250
22. Brooks J, Fuller C, Kemp S, Reddin D (2006) Incidence, risk, and prevention of hamstring muscle injuries in professional rugby union. Am J Sports Med 34:1297–1306
23. Gabbe BL, Branson R, Bennell KL (2006) A pilot randomized controlled trial of eccentric exercise to prevent hamstring injuries in community-level Australian football. J Sci Med Sport 9:103–109
24. Holcomb WR, Rubley MD, Lee HJ, Guadagnoli MA (2007) Effect of hamstring-emphasized resistance training on hamstring: quadriceps strength ratios. J Strength Cond Res 21:41–47
25. Arnason A, Andersen TE, Holme I et al (2008) Prevention of hamstring strains in elite soccer: an intervention study. Scand J Med Sci Sport 18(1):40–48
26. Small K, McNaughton L, Greig M et al (2009) Effect of timing of eccentric hamstring strengthening exercises during soccer training: implications for muscle fatigability. J Strength Cond Res 23(4):1077–1083
27. Comfort P, Green CM, Matthews M (2009) Training considerations after hamstring injury in athletes. Strength Cond J 31:68–74
28. Feland JB, Hawks M, Hopkins JT, Hunter I, Johnson AW, Eggett DL (2010) Whole body vibration as an adjunct to static stretching. Int J Sports Med 31(8):584–589
29. Houston MN, Hodson VE, Adams KKE, Hoch JM (2015) The effectiveness of whole-body-vibration training in improving hamstring flexibility in physically active adults. J Sport Rehabil 24(1):77–82
30. Rittweger J, Mutschelknauss M, Felsenberg D (2003) Acute changes in neuromuscular excitability after exhaustive whole body vibration exercise as compared to exhaustion by squatting exercise. Clin Physiol Funct Imaging 23(2):81–86
31. Bisciotti GN (2005) Aspetti neurofisiologici dell'allenamento vibratorio. Sport e Medicina 2:17–29
32. Sanchez JM (2006) Personal communications

Chapter 9
Pes Anserine Tendinopathy

S. Lupo and Gian Nicola Bisciotti

Abstract Pes anserine tendinopathy can hit sartorius, gracilis, and semitendinosus muscle tendons in their insertion area. Overweight, biomechanical overburden, and improper posture could predispose to this pathology. In fact they provoke excessive friction on the common tendon insertion and underlying bursa that may cause overload work for these muscles and lead to inflammation. This pathology occurs mainly to long-distance runners, young athletes (because of their premature beginning of the sport practice), and especially in women. Symptoms consist in strong pain and burning sensation underneath and inside the knee, where pes anserine tendons insert. In most cases, tendinopathy is provoked by continual mechanical stress causing repeated microtraumas. Therapy consists in rest and appropriate therapeutic and physiotherapeutic treatments.

9.1 Introduction

The pes anserine (PA) or goose's foot is formed by the tendinous insertion of the sartorius (SA), gracilis (GR), and semitendinosus (ST) muscles (Fig. 9.1). This relative strange name of goose's foot is due to the fact that the three muscles attaching to the medial side of tibia form a shape reminiscent of a goose's foot. PA is a structure clinically important in the reconstructive surgery; in fact PA tendons are commonly used as autografts in ligamentous reconstruction of the

S. Lupo (✉)
Istituto di Medicina e Scienza dello Sport, Rome, Italy
e-mail: medicinasport@sportmedicina.com

G.N. Bisciotti
Qatar Orthopaedic and Sport Medicine Hospital, FIFA Center of Excellence, Doha, Qatar
e-mail: bisciotti@libero.it

G.N. Bisciotti, P. Volpi (eds.), *The Lower Limb Tendinopathies*,
Sports and Traumatology, DOI 10.1007/978-3-319-33234-5_9

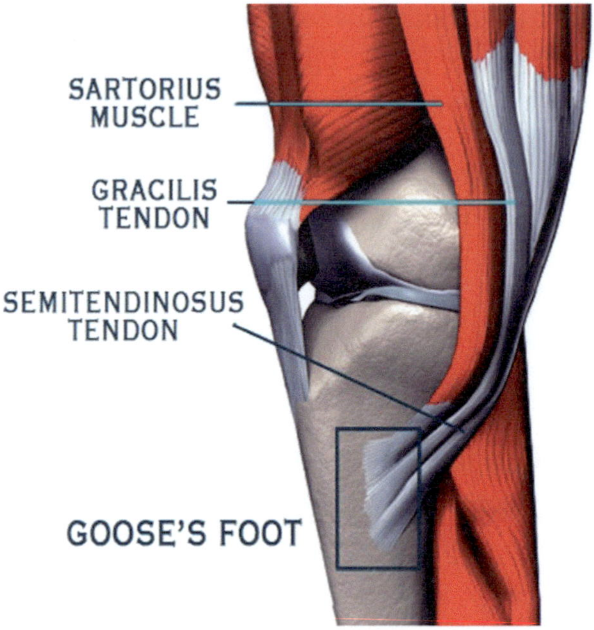

Fig. 9.1 The insertion of sartorius, gracilis, and semitendinosus muscles in the medial area of the knee creates a structure that looks like a goose's foot (after whom it is named)

knees [1, 2]. Studies on cadavers have shown that the SA tendon fascia is intimately attached to the superficial fascial layer; on the contrary the GR and ST tendons are located in the deep surface of the superficial fascial layer over the medial aspect of the tibia [3]. PA presents a bursa, the anserine bursa (AB), that is located at the upper medial aspect of the tibia, in correspondence of the insertion of the conjoined tendon of the PA muscles. Some study [1] reported the presence of accessory bands in gracilis and semitendinosus tendons. The muscle forming PA are main flexors and internally rotators of the knee [4]. In particular SA muscle flexes, abducts, and externally rotates the thigh, while in knee-flexed position flexes and internally rotates the leg (Fig. 9.2). The ST muscle flexes and internally rotates the leg (in a knee-flexed position), extends, and abducts the thigh (Fig. 9.3). The GA muscle adducts and flexes the thigh and flexes and internally rotates the leg (Fig. 9.4).

9.2 Etiopathogenesis of PA Tendinopathy

The first description about PA tendinopathy that we can find in literature dates back to 1937, in that year Moschcowitz [5] described medial knee pain in a female population. The observed patients reported pain when going downstairs

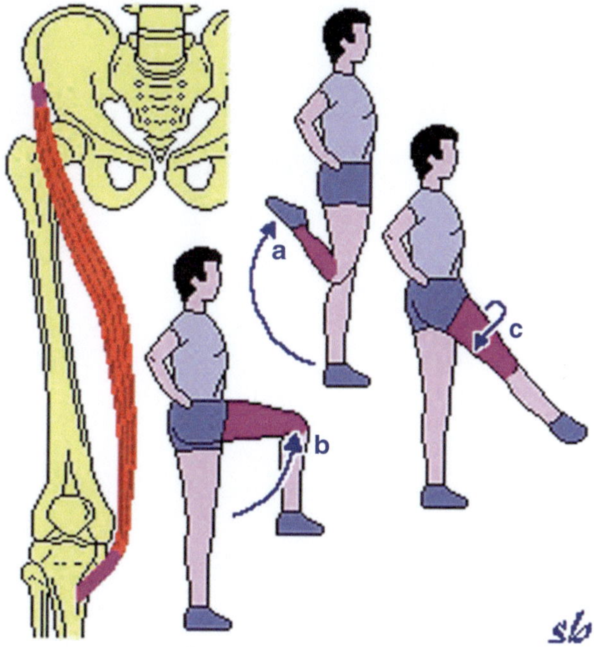

Fig. 9.2 Sartorius muscle flexes (**a**), abducts (**b**), and externally rotates the thigh (**c**), while in knee-flexed position flexes and internally rotates the leg

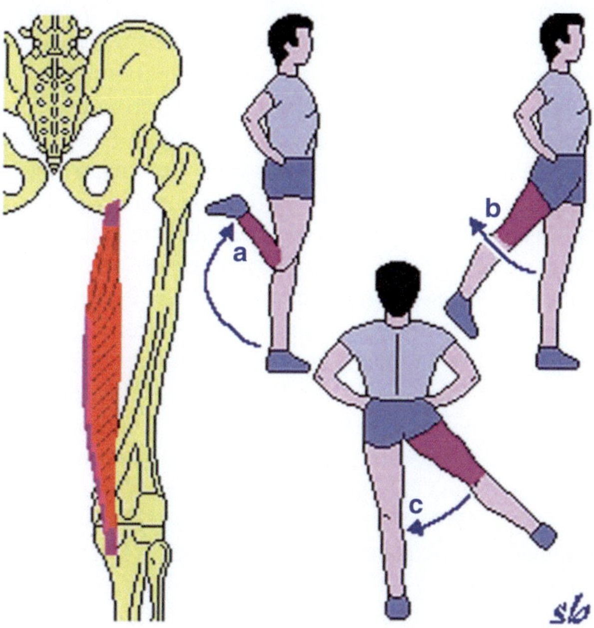

Fig. 9.3 Semitendinosus muscle flexes (**a**) and internally rotates the leg (**b**) (in a knee-flexed position) and extends and abducts the thigh (**c**)

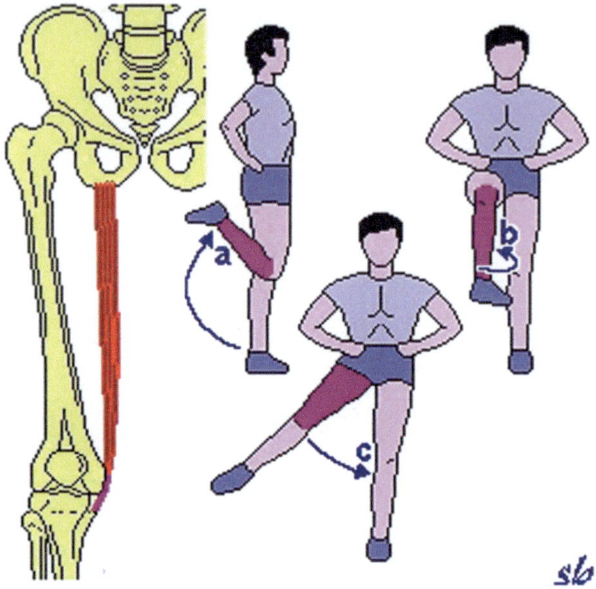

Fig. 9.4 The gracilis muscle adducts and flexes the thigh and flexes and internally rotates the leg

or upstairs, upon rising from a chair, or referred difficulty when flexing the knee. PA tendinopathy is a degenerative condition that can hit these tendons in their insertion area, and it is often linked with AB bursitis. The causes of onset of this pathology may be of intrinsic and extrinsic origin; between the intrinsic causes, we can remember the overweight, a malalignment of the knee, in particular a valgus knee, flatfoot, and postural alteration especially of the pelvis. All these condition may cause an excessive friction on the common tendon insertion [6, 7]. Also diabetes mellitus is known as a predisposing factor [8]. Cases of chronic bursitis concerning AB are well documented in patients with rheumatoid arthritis and osteoarthritis [6, 9, 10]. The intrinsic causes include retraction of posterior thigh muscles, bone exostosis, irritation of the suprapatellar plica, damage to the medial meniscus, and infection [11]. The extrinsic causes are mainly represented by an increase of overuse or trauma as often happens in sport [7]. This pathology occurs mainly in long-distance runners or to young athletes, in this case probably because of their premature beginning of the sport practice [12]. Female gender seems to be more likely to develop PA tendinopathy. This greater predisposition in women is probably due to the fact that women have a wider pelvis, resulting in greater knee Q angle value which leads to more pressure in the area of insertion of the PA [13–15]. In effect, AB bursitis is more common in overweight females with osteoarthritis of the knees [13–15]. In literature we can find several studies based on different imaging modalities focused on the identification if the patients affected by PA tendinopathy suffer only for tendinopathy or from bursitis of AB or both [16–18]. In effect little is known regarding the anatomical structural defect that may be responsible for this pathology. For this reason there is in literature a lack of consensus and some controversies that have led some authors to suggest the term "anserine syndrome" for this specific condition [9]. As of our knowledge until today, no prospective study based on determination whether these patients really suffer from tendinopathy or bursitis or both has been undertaken.

9.3 Clinical Evaluation

Usually the inflammation often comes out after biomechanical overuse, with pain and burning sensation, in the lower internal part of the knee, where PA tendons insert. Symptoms may be particularly evident also in daily leaving activities as going up and down the stairs, or sometimes the pain appears strongly after the patient has been seated a lot and he stands up. Rarely it is possible that an edema appears on PA level, especially if simultaneously there is an AB bursitis. The inflammatory pain persists even at rest; sometimes burning sensation appears during the night, impeding the patient from falling asleep [9]. Diagnosis is imminently clinical also if the history of the patient can be of great help. Patient's history, who complains pain in the medial part of the knee in case of sedentary subject, especially if they are overweight, is often correlated with signs of degenerative joint disease. On the contrary patient's history in case of athlete is often correlated with an overload situation. The clinical evaluation is based on the deep palpation of the affected area; also it is important to note that 30 % of asymptomatic individuals experience pain during deep palpation of the medial area of the knee [7]. Differential diagnosis is based on lesions at the medial meniscus, L3-L4 radiculopathy, lesions at medial collateral ligament, panniculitis, suprapatellar bursitis, prepatellar bursitis, synovial osteochondromatosis, malignant tumors (fibrous histiocytoma, liposarcoma, and synovial sarcoma), varicose popliteal vein, popliteal aneurysm, infectious complication of surgical procedure, osteonecrosis affecting the medial tibial plateau, patellofemoral syndrome, patellar chondromalacia, recurring patellar subluxation, and direct trauma. Frequently, pain in the anserine region is part of the fibromyalgia syndrome [19]. Another differential diagnosis to consider is represented by semimembranosus bursitis (SB). SB, also called semimembranosus tibial collateral ligament bursitis, is an inflammatory process of the semimembranosus bursa that is within the superficial and deep layers of the medial collateral ligament and involves the anterosuperior margin of the semimembranosus tendon [20]. In the same manner, we must also consider iliotibial bursitis (IB) as differential diagnosis. The ITB is an inflammatory process regarding the iliotibial bursa. The iliotibial bursa is located between the distal portion of the iliotibial band (near its insertion in the Gerdy tuberculum) and the adjacent tibial surface. The ITB can be associated with iliotibial tendinitis and it is usually due to overload and varus stress [21].

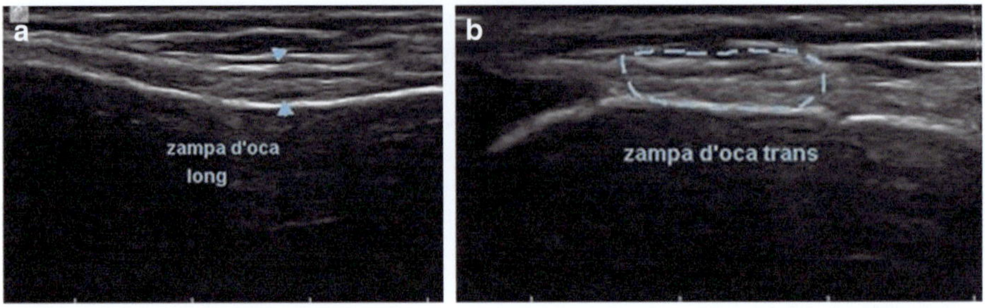

Fig. 9.5 Ultrasound longitudinal examination (**a**) and axial examination (**b**) of pes anserine in normal anatomical situation

9.4 Imaging Assessment

Also if the diagnosis is imminently clinical, this latter can be corroborated by imaging exams. In this regard it is important to remember that relatively few studies using imaging exams assessed the morphological characteristics of the PA tendons insertion and respective AB in a patient population that has clinical diagnosis of anserine syndrome [6, 16, 17, 22–25]. These studies showed substantially that only a minority of patients with clinical diagnosis of anserine syndrome have compatible anatomical ultrasound changes. Then, since the ultrasound might not detect the abnormalities produced by a PA tendinopathy and/or AB bursitis, MRI might present a contribution. In any case the current literature shows that ultrasound, CT, and MRI findings usually do not allow the identification of anatomical structure responsible for the symptoms in PA tendinopathy and/or AB bursitis. In Fig. 9.5 we report a PA ultrasound normal anatomical situation.

9.5 Conservative Treatment

The treatment starts, first of all, with an initial period of rest and abstinence from the daily activities potentially dangerous. In overweight subjects it is very important to lose weight. The initial treatment should include resting and cryotherapy. The use of a pillow between the thighs at nighttimes is strongly recommended. Physiotherapy has an important role in the treatment of PA tendinopathy and AB bursitis. The use of ultrasound has been documented as effective in the reduction of the inflammatory process [26]. Stretching of SA, GR, and ST is strongly recommended. In effect an improvement in flexibility obtainable through a systematic program of passive and active stretching can promote an important reduction in the tension on the anserine bursa [27]. The medical treatment involves the use of FANS. Another possible option is represented by the injection of local anesthetic associated with corticosteroids in the AB in cases of proven AB bursitis. Some authors suggest the use of 20–40 mg of methylprednisolone [26, 28, 29]; triamcinolone, 20–40 mg; or betamethasone, 6 mg [30]. In any case no more than three infiltrations should be done over a 1-year period; furthermore the interval time between infiltrations should be greater than 1 month. It is important to note that rarely the patients who do not show any positive response to an initial infiltration respond to repeated infiltrations. Some studies have demonstrated that infiltration with corticosteroids represent a valid good option in well-selected patients [9, 31, 32]. However, it is important to note that cortisone injections are not without risk that is represented by atrophy of the subcutaneous tissue, skin depigmentation, and tendon rupture [30, 33].

9.6 Surgical Treatment

Surgical treatment is rare and obviously is indicated in case of failure of the conservative treatment. In the case of AB bursitis, it consists in an incision followed by drainage of the distended bursa; generally this simple surgical act can provide improvement of symptom [9, 26, 28, 34].

In cases of exostosis, the surgery includes excision of the bursa and the removal of any bony exostosis [34]. However, in literature we can find the description of the cases in which the removal of the bursa was necessary [11]. In case of important tendinopathy associated with AB bursitis, arthroscopic debridement can be considered [35].

9.7 Conclusions

Many patients that show pain in the medial compartment of the knee receive the diagnosis of PA tendinopathy, AB bursitis, or both these conditions. However, the diagnosis is based only on the presence of pain on palpation in the anatomic site, and when patients are submitted to imaging exams these last do not confirm the clinical diagnosis. Very often in effect, especially in certain patients (i.e., female patients in overweight), a panniculitis of the fat tissue of the medial compartment can be exchanged with PA tendinopathy or AB bursitis. Instead in the case of osteoarthrosis, it is very important to underline that both PA tendinopathy and AB bursitis must be considered as secondary or associated pathology. It is therefore very likely that a true PA tendinopathy and AB bursitis (i.e., that can be considered as primary pathology) can be found only in athletes.

References

1. Candal-Couto JJ, Deehan DJ (2003) The accessory bands of Gracilis and Semitendinosus: an anatomical study. Knee 10:325–328. 2
2. Mochizuki T, Akita K, Muneta T, Sato T (2004) Pes anserinus: layered supportive structure on the medial side of the knee. Clin Anat 17:50–54
3. LaPrade RF, Engebretsen AH, Ly TV, Johansen S, Wentorf FA, Engebretsen L (2007) The anatomy of the medial part of the knee. J Bone Joint Surg Am 89:2000–2010

4. Lee JH, Kim KJ, Jeong YG, Lee NS, Han SY, Lee CG, Kim KY, Han SH (2014) Pes anserinus and anserine bursa: anatomical study. Anat Cell Biol 47(2):127–131
5. Moschcowitz E (1937) Bursitis of sartorius bursa: an undescribed malady simulating chronic arthritis. JAMA 109:1362–1366
6. Rennie WJ, Saifuddin A (2005) Pes anserine bursitis: incidence in symptomatic knees and clinical presentation. Skeletal Radiol 34:395–398
7. Helfenstein M Jr, Kuromoto J (2010) Anserine syndrome. Rev Bras Reumatol 50(3):313–327
8. Cohen SE, Mahul O, Meir R (1997) Anserine bursitis and non-insulin dependent diabetes mellitus. J Rheumatol 24:2162–2165
9. Larsson LG, Baum J (1986) The syndromes of bursitis. Bull Rheum Dis 36:1–8
10. Larsson LG, Baum J (1985) The syndrome of anserine bursitis: an overlooked diagnosis. Arthritis Rheum 28:1062–1065
11. Huang TW, Wang CJ, Huang SC (2003) Polyethylene-induced pes anserinus bursitis mimicking and infected total knee arthroplasty. J Arthroplasty 18:383–386
12. Hall R, Barber Foss K, Hewett TE, Myer GD (2015) Sports specialization is associated with an increased risk of developing anterior knee pain in adolescent female athletes. J Sport Rehabil 24:31–35
13. Handy JR (1997) Anserine bursitis: a brief review. South Med J 90:376–377
14. Gnanadesigan N, Smith RL (2003) Knee pain: osteoarthritis or anserine bursitis? J Am Med Dir Assoc 4:164–166
15. Nemegyei A, Jose MD, Canoso JJ (2004) Evidence-based soft tissue rheumatology IV: anserine bursitis. J Clin Rheumatol 10:205–206
16. Uson J, Aguado P, Bernad M, Mayordomo L, Naredo E, Balsa A et al (2000) Pes anserinus tendino-bursitis: what are we talking about? Scand J Rheumatol 29:184–186
17. Hill CL, Gale DR, Chasson CE (2003) Periarticular lesions detected on magnetic resonance imaging: prevalence in knees with and without symptoms. Arthr Rheum 48:2836–2844
18. Unlu Z, Ozmen B, Taethan S, Boyvoda S, Goktan C (2003) Ultrasonographic evaluation of pes anserinus tendino-bursitis in patients with type 2 diabetes mellitus. J Rheumatol 30:352–354. 21
19. Genç H, Saracoğlu M, Duyur B, Erdem HR (2003) The role of tendinitis in fibromyalgia syndrome. Yonsei Med J 44(4):619–622
20. Demeyere N, De Maeseneer M, Van Roy P, Osteaux M, Shahabpour M (2003) Imaging of semimembranosus bursitis: MR findings in three patients and anatomical study. JBR-BTR 86(6):332–334
21. Hariri S, Savidge ET, Reinold MM, Zachazewski J, Gill TJ (2009) Treatment of recalcitrant iliotibial band friction syndrome with open iliotibial band bursectomy: indications, technique, and clinical outcomes. Am J Sports Med 37(7):1417–1424
22. Hall FM, Joffe N (1988) CT imaging of the anserine bursa. Am J Roentgenol 150:1107–1108
23. Forbes JR, Helms CA, Janzen DL (1995) Acute pes anserine bursitis: MR imaging. Radiology 194:525–527. 24
24. Muchnick J, Sundaram M (1997) Radiologic case study. Orthopedics 20:1092–1094. 25
25. Koh WL, Kwek JW, Quek ST, Peh WCG (2002) Clinics in diagnostic imaging. Singapore Med J 43:485–491. 26
26. Brookler MI, Mongan ES (1973) Anserine bursitis: a treatable cause of knee pain in patients with degenerative arthritis. Calif Med 119:8–10
27. Helfenstein M Jr, Kuromoto J (2010) Anserine syndrome. Bras J Rheumatol 50(3):313–327
28. Abeles M (1983) Osteoarthritis of the knee: anserine bursitis as an extraarticular cause of pain. Clin Res 31:4471–4476
29. O'Donoghue DH (1987) Injuries of the knee. In: O'Donoghue DH (ed) Treatment of injuries to athletes, 4th edn. W.B. Saunders, Philadelphia, pp 470–471
30. Glencross PM, Little JP (2009) Pes anserine bursitis. eMedicine Journal. http://emedicine.medscape.com/article/308694-treatment. Atualizado em 10 setembro 2009
31. Calvo-Alén J, Rua-Figueroa I, Erausquin C (1993) Tratamiento de las bursitis anserina: infiltración local com corticoides frente a AINE: estudo prospectivo. Rev Esp Reumatol 20:13–15. 39

32. Kang I (2000) Anserine bursitis in patients with osteoarthritis of the knee. South Med J 93:207–209
33. Saunders S, Cameron G (1997) Injection techniques in orthopedic and sports medicine, 1st edn. W.B. Saunders, Philadelphia, pp 8–9
34. Zeiss J, Coombs R, Booth R, Saddemi S (1993) Chronic bursitis presenting as a mass in the pes anserine bursa: MR diagnosis. J Comput Assist Tomogr 17:137–141
35. Yan C, Chen B, Shao D, Kang H, Liu H, Wang S, Li J (2009) Treatment of Pes anserinus bursitis with debridement under arthroscopy. Zhongguo Xiu Fu Chong Jian Wai Ke Za Zhi 23(9):1045–1048

Chapter 10
Achilles Tendinopathy

Nicola Maffulli, Alessio Giai Via, and Francesco Oliva

Abstract Achilles tendinopathy is a common cause of disability. Despite the economic and social relevance of the problem, the causes and mechanisms of Achilles tendinopathy remain unclear. Tendon vascularity, gastrocnemius-soleus dysfunction, age, sex, body weight and height, pes cavus, and lateral ankle instability are considered common risk factors. Currently, intratendinous degenerative changes are considered responsible for tendinopathy and symptoms. Although Achilles tendinopathy has been extensively studied, there is a clear lack of properly conducted scientific research to clarify the optimal management option. The management of Achilles tendinopathy lacks evidence-based support, and patients are at risk of long-term morbidity with unpredictable clinical outcome. Most patients respond to conservative management. Eccentric exercises and shockwave provide excellent clinical results both in athletic and sedentary patients, with no reported adverse effects. However, in about 20–45 % of cases, patients do not respond well to conservative treatment, and they need surgery. Both minimally invasive and open surgeries have been described with similar results.

N. Maffulli, MD, PhD, FRCP, FRCS (✉)
Department of Musculoskeletal Disorders, School of Medicine and Surgery,
University of Salerno, Salerno, Italy

Barts and the London School of Medicine and Dentistry,
Centre for Sports and Exercise Medicine,
Mary University of London, Mile End Hospital,
275 Bancroft Road, London E1 4DG, UK
e-mail: n.maffulli@qmul.ac.uk; n.maffulli@keele.ac.uk

A. Giai Via, MD • F. Oliva, MD, PhD
Department of Orthopaedic and Traumatology,
University of Rome "Tor Vergata", School of Medicine,
Viale Oxford 81, 00133 Rome, Italy
e-mail: alessiogiaivia@hotmail.it; olivafrancesco@hotmail.com

G.N. Bisciotti, P. Volpi (eds.), *The Lower Limb Tendinopathies*,
Sports and Traumatology, DOI 10.1007/978-3-319-33234-5_10

10.1 Introduction

Achilles tendinopathy (AT) is characterized by pain, swelling, impaired performance ability, and pathologic changes in and around the tendon. In chronic AT, symptoms have been present longer than 6 months [1]. The incidence has risen in the past three decades as a result of greater participation in sporting activities. AT is estimated to occur in 7–9 % of top-level runners. A tenfold increase in Achilles tendon injuries has been reported in runners compared to age-matched controls [2]. AT is also common in individuals participating in racquet sports, track and field, volleyball, and soccer. However, the condition is not confined to athletes because 30 % of patients have a sedentary lifestyle [3].

10.2 Etiopathogenesis of Achilles Tendinopathy

The etiopathogenesis of AT remains unclear. It is currently considered multifactorial, and the interaction between extrinsic and intrinsic factors has been postulated [1]. Extrinsic factors such as increased frequency and duration of training have been associated with AT. Changes in training pattern, poor technique, previous injuries, footwear, and environmental factors such as training on hard, slippery, or slanting surfaces may predispose athletes to tendinopathy [4]. However, a retrospective study showed that tendinopathy was not necessarily associated with the level of physical activity [5]. Some drugs and antibiotics such as fluoroquinolones and corticosteroids have been recognized as risk factors of tendinopathy and Achilles tendon ruptures. Ciprofloxacin causes enhanced interleukin-1b-mediated MMP3 release, inhibits tenocytes proliferation, and, like corticosteroids, reduces collagen and matrix synthesis [6].

Intrinsic factors include lower limb anatomy, biomechanics, previous injuries, gender, age, metabolic disorders, and systemic diseases. Lower limb alignment and biomechanical faults are claimed to play a causative role in two-thirds of athletes with Achilles tendon disorders. Malalignment and hyperpronation impose excessive strain on the Achilles tendon, and hyperpronation of the foot has been linked with an increased incidence of AT [7].

The incidence of tendinopathy is lower in women than men, and estrogen levels might play an important role in tendon homeostasis [6]. Women showed a lower risk of tendinopathy during premenopausal years than man, but, after menopause, this risk increases [8]. Postmenopausal estrogen deficiency seems to downregulate collagen turnover and to decrease elasticity in tendon. An animal study showed poorer Achilles tendon healing in estrogen-deficient rats compared to controls [9], and Cook et al. reported that the Achilles tendon health of women using hormone replacement therapy was better than the controls [10]. However, little is known about the effect of estrogen on tenocytes. A recent in vitro study showed that proliferation and tenocytes biosynthesis are negatively affected by age and estrogen deficiency [11]. Tenocytes from ovariectomized and old rats showed a significantly lower proliferation rate, a decreased collagen type I synthesis, and overexpression of MMPs compared to young controls, showing that aging and, more significantly, estrogen levels may affect tendon metabolism and healing.

Connective tissue aging is associated with compromised tissue function, increased susceptibility to injury, and reduced healing capacity. This has been partly attributed to collagen cross-linking by advanced glycation end products (AGEs) that accumulate with both age and chronic diseases, in particular diabetes mellitus [12]. Protein glycation is a spontaneous reaction depending on the degree and duration of hyperglycemia, the half-life of the protein, and permeability of the tissue to free glucose. Glycated proteins can undergo further reactions giving rise to poorly characterized structures called advanced glycation end products (AGEs). AGEs are complex, heterogeneous molecules that cause protein cross-linking, which alter physical characteristics of collagen fibers, and they may affect the tendon properties [13]. The effects of AGEs on the mechanical properties of tendon collagen fiber have been recently studied in a rat model [14]. The formation of AGEs would change the way tendon reacts to loading, in particular significantly reducing collagen fiber sliding. On the other hand, tendons try to compensate this loss of function by increasing collagen fiber stretch which may have potentially important implications for predisposing collagen fibrils to damage during everyday use. Tissue stiffness does not appear to be significantly affected. Therefore, physiological loads in aged and diabetic tendons could involve fiber "overstretching" that leads to accelerated accumulation of damage.

The relationship between thyroid disorders and joint pain has been suspected since the late 1920s [15], but it has not been systematically investigated. Thyroid hormones (THs) play an essential role in the development and metabolism of many tissues. Thyroxine (T4) is important for both collagen synthesis and extracellular matrix (ECM) metabolism. A recent study demonstrates that TH nuclear receptors are present on tenocytes and that, in vitro, THs enhance tenocytes growth and counteract apoptosis in healthy tenocytes isolated from tendon in a dose- and time-dependent manner [16]. This may be reason why the incidence of tendon tears is higher in patients affected by hypothyroidism. [17].

The physiopathology of tendinopathy in obese patients has yet to be understood, but some studies show that obesity may affect tendon health and reduce its healing ability [18]. Many authors consider obesity as a risk factor for tendons injury [19]. Anatomic studies show that Achilles tendons are significantly thicker in obese individuals than in a control group [20], and ultrasonography showed thicker and hypoechogenic tendons in obese subjects compared to normal individuals [21]. Histological changes have been observed in animal studies. Lipid drops accumulate in the extracellular matrix [22], and disorganized collagen fibrils are observed at transmission electron microscopy in the tendon ECM of obese animals [23]. Low levels of glycosaminoglycans (chondroitin and dermatan sulfate), which play an important role in the regulation of the ECM and collagen fibrillogenesis, have been detected, and they may be responsible for the inadequate deposition and organization of collagen fibrils [24]. Finally, obesity is frequently associated with other pathologies, such as diabetes mellitus and insulin resistance, which may also play a role in tendon pathology.

Many studies currently advocate the importance of extracellular matrix (ECM) for the homeostasis of connective tissue, and its physiological and pathological modifications seem the most important intrinsic factors involved in tendinopathies and tendons ruptures [25]. The turnover of ECM in normal tendons is mediated by matrix metalloproteinases (MMPs) [26], MMP-1, MMP-2, and MMP-3 [27]. They are able to denature collagen type I. After tendon rupture, the activity of MMP-1 increases, while a reduction of MMP-2 and MMP-3 has been showed [28]. An increase in MMP-1 activity and degradation of the collagen type I network is a potential cause of the weakening of the tendon, and it may contribute to tendinopathy and rupture. These findings may represent a failure of the normal matrix remodeling process.

Transglutaminases (TGs) are also implicated in the formation of hard tissue development, matrix maturation, and mineralization [29]. Nine different TGs have been found in mammalian. TG2, also known as tissue transglutaminase, is widely distributed within many connective tissues, and it is implicated in organogenesis, tissue repair, and tissue stabilization. An animal model showed a reduction of TG2 protein expression in tendinopathic supraspinatus tendons [30]. TGs are important in maintaining the structural integrity of tendons thanks to their mechanical or cross-linking function in normal condition, and the fall of TG2 may mean the exhaustion of the reparative capabilities of the tendon.

10.3 Achilles Tendinopathy: Why Painful?

Although significant advances have been made in understanding its pathogenesis, relatively little is known about the source of pain associated with AT. Intratendinous degenerative changes are believed to be the responsible of symptoms. However, intratendinous degenerative changes often occur without symptoms. This is the reason why Achilles tendon rupture often occurs without previous symptoms: histopathological changes alone cannot be the only reason for pain. Recent research identified the peripheral and central pain processing pathways as an important factor in the pathogenesis of painful human tendinopathy, and changes in the peripheral neuronal phenotype may be the primary source of pain [31]. Peripheral neuronal phenotype refers to specific characteristics of the peripheral nervous system including nerves, neuronal mediators, and receptors.

Healthy tendons are relatively aneuronal. The neural supply to the Achilles tendon and the surrounding paratenon is provided by nerves from the attaching muscles and by small fasciculi from cutaneous nerves, in particular the sural nerve [32], but they do not have a rich nervous supply [33]. Indeed, chronic painful tendons present ingrowth of new nerve fibers accompanying the peritendinous neovascularization from the paratenon into the tendon proper [33]. Alfredson et al. demonstrated increased neural ingrowth in AT versus control [34]. The authors found strong evidence of an upregulation of the glutaminergic system in painful human tendinopathy, and weaker, but still suggestive, evidence that changes in the peripheral neuronal phenotype were related to variations in pain among patients. Glutamate is a key metabolite and neurotransmitter involved in the transmission of pain. Glutamate NMDAR1 receptors have been frequently noted in morphologically altered tenocytes in tendon tissue proper and in the peritendinous connective tissue [35]. There is also some evidence for upregulation of the substance P/CGRP system, which has been linked with increased nociception in both animal models and human disease [31]. Substance P is also associated with vasodilation and stimulates the proliferation of fibroblasts [36], possibly causing some of the morphologic changes in AT.

10.4 Clinical Aspects of Achilles Tendinopathy

Clinical history and examination are essential for diagnosis. A detailed history helps to identify the onset and possible contributing factors. Pain is the main symptom. Pain is usually referred 2–6 cm proximally to the tendon insertion [33]. Initially, pain occurs at the beginning and a short while after the end of a training session with a period of diminished discomfort in between. Runner typically report pain at the beginning ad at the end of the training session, with a pain-free period in the central part [37], but as the pathological process progresses, pain may occur during the entire exercise session. In severe cases, it may interfere with activities of daily living. A good correlation between severity of symptoms and morning stiffness has been reported [38].

On examination, both lower limbs should be exposed, and the patent should be examined standing and prone. The lower limb should be inspected for malalignment, deformities, muscular hypotrophy, and previous scars. The Achilles tendon should be palpated for tenderness, increased local temperature, thickening, and crepitation (Fig. 10.1).

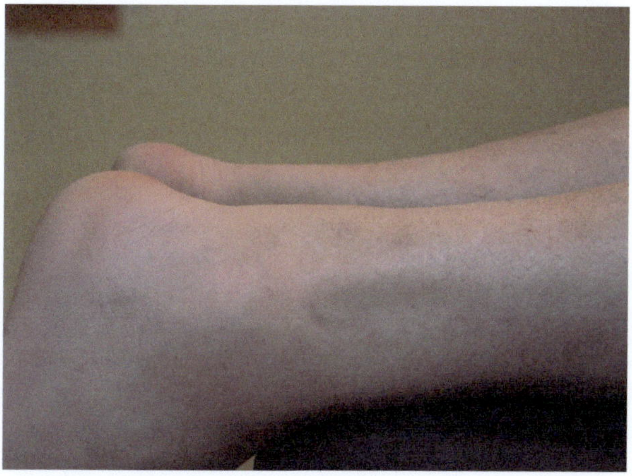

Fig. 10.1 Tendinopathy of the right Achilles tendon

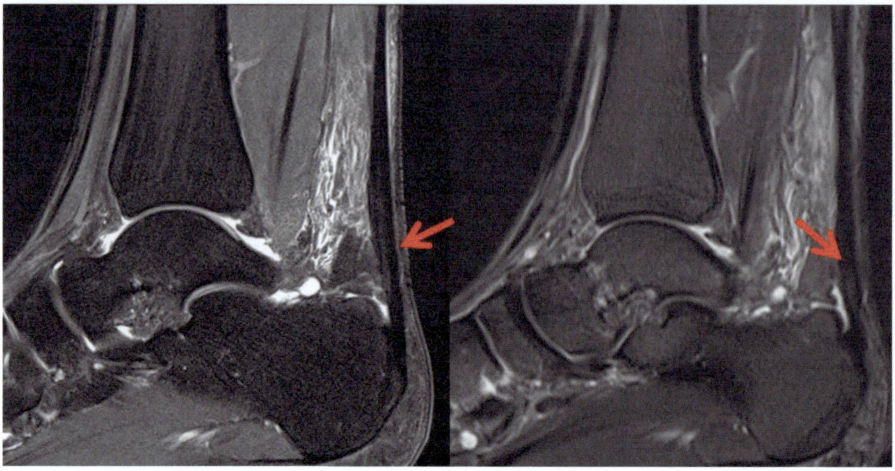

Fig. 10.2 MRI imaging of Achilles tendinopathy (*arrow*)

Plain radiography can be used to diagnose associated bony abnormalities or a calcific tendinopathy [39]. Ultrasound, despite being operator dependent, correlates well with the histopathologic findings, and it is an effective imaging method [40]. MRI provides extensive information on the internal morphology of the tendon and the surrounding structures (Fig. 10.2) and is useful in evaluating the various stages of AT and in differentiating between paratendinopathy and tendinopathy. Areas of mucoid degeneration are shown on MRI as a zone of high signal intensity on T1- and T2-weighted images [41]. Thickening of the Achilles tendon can be easily demonstrated at both MR and ultrasound.

10.5 Prevention of Achilles Tendinopathy

As the management of AT lacks evidence-based support, patients are often at risk of long-term morbidity with unpredictable clinical outcome. The rehabilitation protocols and treatments are long and time consuming. For these reasons, exercise programs which aim to prevent AT are important. However, even if various preventive interventions protocols have been described, there is still little evidence on their effectiveness. A recent systematic review of literature tried to report the current evidence about preventive exercise programs for tendinopathies [42]. Stretching exercise is an empirically accepted and commonly used method to prevent sports injuries and tendinopathy. However, there is no evidence for a positive effect of stretching exercises alone [42–44]. But, when stretching exercises were used together with exercise programs, a significant reduction in the incidence of tendinopathy was reported. Kraemer and Knobloch found that a program that included soccer-specific balance training can significantly reduce the incidence of patellar and Achilles tendinopathy [45]. They also found a dose-effect relationship between duration of balance training and injury incidence.

In addition to stretch and exercise interventions, shoe adaptations such as orthoses are used in the prevention and treatment of lower extremity tendinopathies. Three articles focused on the use of orthoses are available in current literature [46–48], but only House and colleagues found a statistically significant difference with the use of shock-absorbing insoles on the incidence of AT in a military population [49].

Cook et al. [10] studied the effects of activity levels and hormonal status on Achilles tendon structure in asymptomatic postmenopausal women. They found that active postmenopausal women had a greater prevalence of tendon abnormalities and thicker Achilles tendons than inactive women and that hormone replacement therapy seems to reduce the risk for structural Achilles tendon changes in this group of women.

10.6 Conservative Treatment of Achilles Tendinopathy

Many different conservative treatments as physical therapy, rest, training modification, splintage, taping, cryotherapy, electrotherapy, shock wave therapy, hyperthermia, pharmaceutical agents such as NSAIDs, and various peritendinous injections have all been proposed. Managements that have been investigated with randomized controlled trials include nonsteroidal anti-inflammatory medication, eccentric exercise, glyceryl trinitrate patches, electrotherapy (microcurrent and microwave), sclerosing injections, and shock wave treatment [49].

Eccentric training was first advocated in the management of tendinopathy over two decades ago by Stanish et al. [50]. The concept of eccentric exercises is based on the structural adaptation of the musculotendinous units. However, the mechanism for the efficacy of eccentric loading is largely unknown. A possible mechanism which seems to enhance tendon healing is mechanical conditioning [51]. Mechanotransduction is the process of a cell converting mechanical stimuli into biochemical signals. Tendon responds to mechanical forces by adapting its metabolism, structural, and mechanical properties [52]. Alfredson et al. reported decrease of neovascularization after an eccentric training intervention at color Doppler sonography [53]. Several studies reported good short- and long-term results after eccentric training superior to controls [53–55]. Significant improvement in patient satisfaction and decreased pain were seen in 60–90 % of patients [56] (Fig. 10.3).

Shock wave therapies (SWTs) are widely used for the management of tendon disorders. Two different types of SWs are used in clinical practice, extracorporeal shockwave therapy (ESWT) and “radial shock wave therapy” (RSWT) or “radial pulse therapy” (RPT). ESWTs are concentrated into small focal areas of 2–8 mm diameter. Ultrasound guide is needed to focus the shock wave, and refocusing of the applicator is periodically necessary. RSWTs are not focused, and, once located, the area to treat is included within the wave propagation area, and they do not need periodical refocusing of the applicator. The disadvantage is that they do not have a penetrating effect on tissue but act superficially. Lohrer et al. reported significant pain reduction and increased functionality in patients with AT who

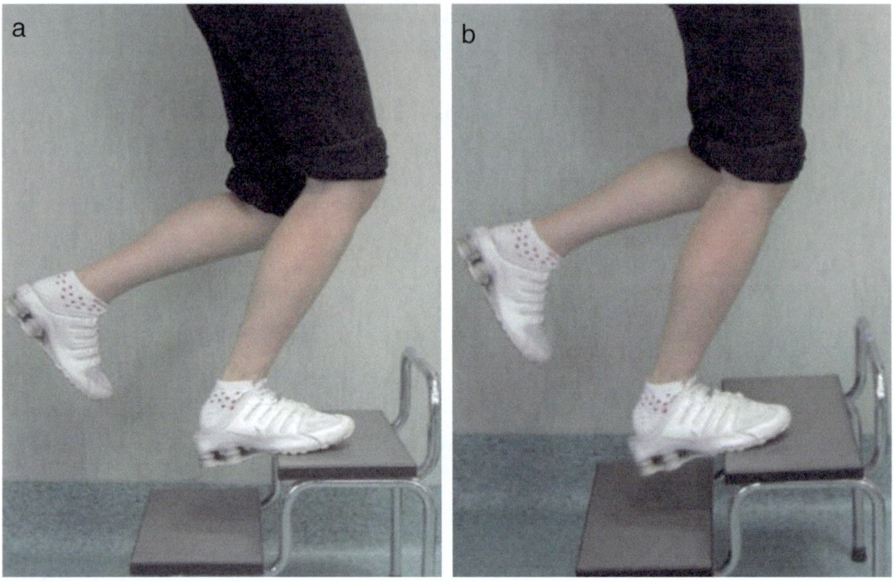

Fig. 10.3 (**a**) Eccentric exercise with the knee straight, to maximize the activation of the gastrocnemius muscle. (**b**) Eccentric exercise with the knee bent, to maximize the activation of the soleus muscle. Please note that, in clinical practice, it is sufficient to undertake the eccentric exercises only with the knee straight

received RSWT [57]. In a small RCT of 39 patients, Peers reported a 77 % success rate at 12-week follow-up [58]. In a RCT, Rompe et al. compared the effectiveness of three management strategies [41]. Group one was treated with eccentric loading exercises, group two was treated with repetitive low energy SWT, and group 3 was treated with a "wait-and-see" approach. At 4 months follow-up, clinical results did not differ significantly between group 1 and 2, but they were significantly better than group 3. A recent systematic review [59] reported some evidence of benefit with high-energy ESWT in midportion AT [60] and lack of benefit of low-dose ESWT [61].

10.7 Minimally Invasive Treatment

Even though open surgery can provide good results, wound complications are frequent. Minimally invasive techniques reduce the risks of infection and wound breakdown and are inexpensive and technically easy to perform. The rationale behind most of these techniques is to break the neovessels and the accompanying nerve supply which may be responsible of pain in most of patients. They can also be associated with other minimally invasive procedures to optimize results, providing great potential for the management of chronic AT.

10.7.1 High-Volume Injections

High-volume image-guided injections (HVIGIs) target the neurovascular bundles growing from the paratenon into the Achilles tendon. Several substances have been injected in and around tendons including normal saline, corticosteroids, and local anesthetics [62, 63]. The injection is performed under ultrasound guidance to avoid intratendinous injections. Patients are allowed to walk on the injected leg immediately, but they are strictly advised to refrain from high-impact activities for 72 h. After this period, they are instructed to restart eccentric loading physiotherapy regime twice daily until they stop their sporting career. Good results have been reported with this technique at short-term follow-up [64]. Platelet-rich plasma injections did not show the expected benefits for AT when administered in randomized controlled trial conditions [65].

10.7.2 Minimally Invasive Achilles Tendon Stripping

The patient is placed prone. Four skin incisions 5 mm length are made, two at the proximal origin of the Achilles tendon, just medial and lateral to the origin of the tendon, and the other two 1 cm distal to the distal end of the tendon insertion on the calcaneus. A mosquito is inserted in the proximal incisions, and the Achilles tendon is freed of the peritendinous adhesions. A number 1 unmounted Ethibond (Ethicon, Somerville, NJ) suture thread is inserted proximally, passing through the two proximal incisions (Fig. 10.4). The Ethibond is retrieved from the distal incisions, over the anterior aspect of the Achilles tendon. Using a gentle seesaw motion, the Ethibond suture thread is made to slide anterior to the tendon (Fig. 10.5), which is stripped and freed from the fat of Kager's triangle (Fig. 10.6).

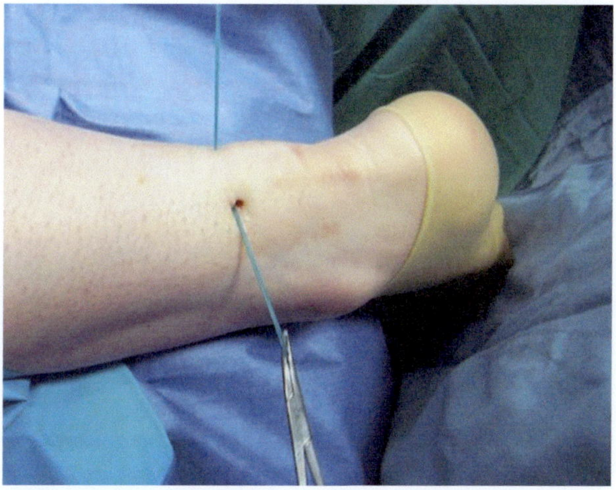

Fig. 10.4 The suture is inserted proximally through the two proximal incisions

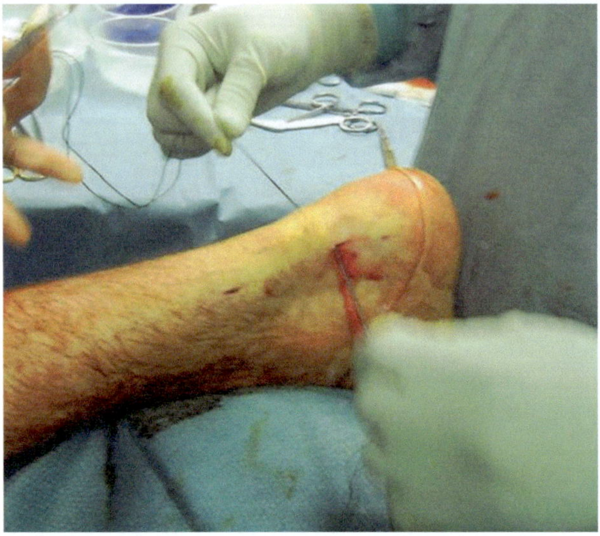

Fig. 10.5 The suture is slid over the anterior aspect of the Achilles tendon with a gentle seesaw motion

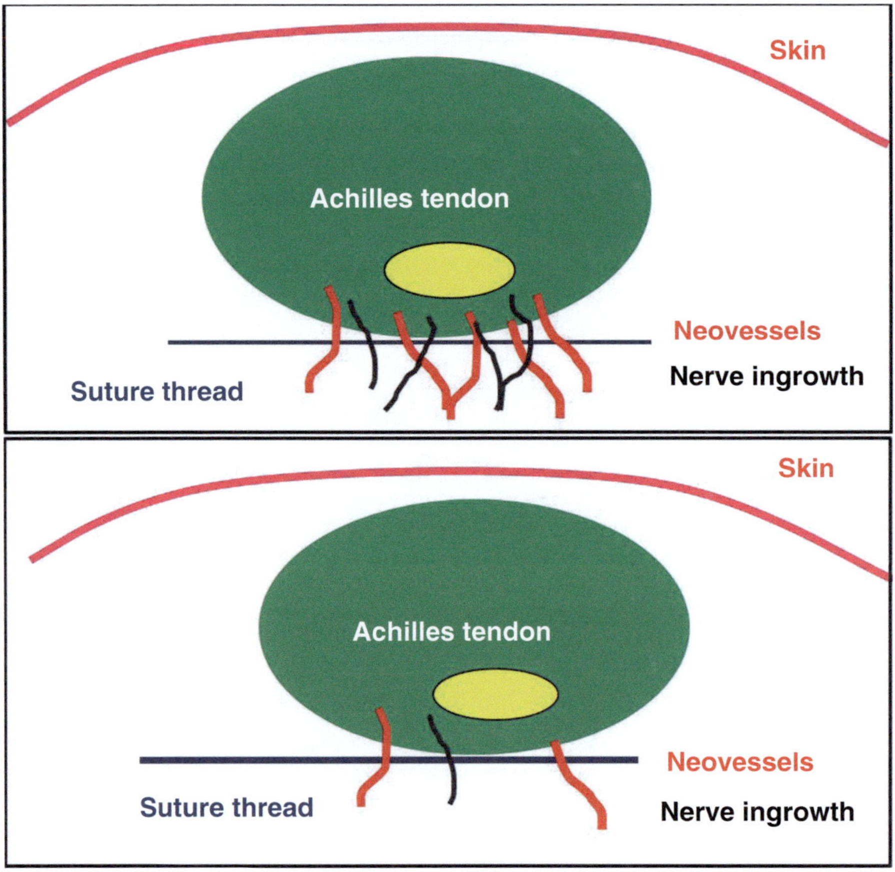

Fig. 10.6 Figure showing the rationale behind minimally invasive Achilles tendon stripping. The suture aim to break vascular and neural ingrowth from the paratenon which is responsible of pain

If necessary, using an 11 blade, longitudinal percutaneous tenotomies parallel to the tendon fibers are made.

Postoperatively, patients are allowed to mobilize fully weight bearing. After 2 weeks, patients start physiotherapy, focusing on proprioception, plantar flexion of the ankle, inversion, and eversion.

10.7.3 Percutaneous Longitudinal Tenotomies

Percutaneous longitudinal tenotomy can be used when there is no paratenon involvement and when the intratendinous lesion is smaller than 2.5 cm. The procedure can be performed under ultrasound guidance [66]. The patient lies prone on the operating table, and a bloodless field is not necessary. The tendon is accurately palpated, and the area of maximum swelling and/or tenderness marked and checked again by US scanning. The skin and the subcutaneous tissues over the Achilles tendon are infiltrated with 10–15 mL of plain 1 % lignocaine. A number 11 surgical scalpel blade is inserted parallel to the long axis of the tendon fibers in the marked area in the center of the area of tendinopathy. The cutting edge of the blade points caudally and penetrates the whole thickness of the tendon (Fig. 10.6). Keeping the blade still, a full passive ankle dorsiflexion movement is produced. The scalpel blade is then retracted to the surface of the tendon, inclined 45° on the sagittal axis, and the blade is inserted medially through the original tenotomy (Fig. 10.7). Keeping the blade still, a full passive ankle flexion is produced. The whole procedure is repeated inclining the blade 45° laterally to the original tenotomy, inserting it laterally through the original tenotomy. Keeping the blade still, a full passive ankle flexion is produced. The blade is then partially retracted to the posterior surface of the Achilles tendon, reversed 180°, so that its cutting edge now points cranially, and the whole procedure repeated, taking care to dorsiflex the ankle passively. Preliminary cadaveric studies showed that a tenotomy 2.8 cm long on average is thus obtained through a stab wound in the main body of the tendon [63].

The patient is operated as day case. Early active dorsi- and plantar flexion of the foot are encouraged. On the second postoperative day, patients are allowed to walk

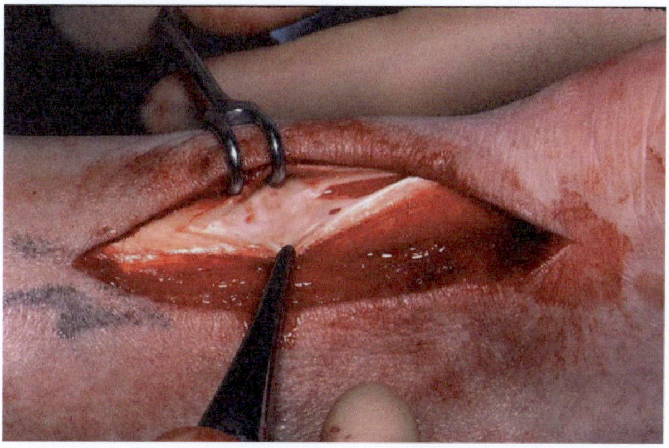

Fig. 10.7 Open excision of degenerated Achilles tendon area

with 2 crutches and weight bearing as able. Stationary bicycling and isometric, concentric, and eccentric strengthening of the calf muscles are started under physiotherapy guidance after 4 weeks. Swimming and water running are encouraged from the second week. Gentle running is started 4–6 weeks after the procedure, and mileage gradually increased.

We reported excellent and good results in 63 % of athletes with unilateral AT treated with ultrasound-guided percutaneous longitudinal tenotomy after failure of conservative management, without experienced significant complications [67].

10.7.4 Open Surgery

Under locoregional or general anesthesia, the patient is placed prone with the ankles clear of the operating table. A tourniquet is applied to the limb to be operated on. The incision is made on the medial side of the tendon to avoid injury to the sural nerve and short saphenous vein. The skin edge of the incision should be handled with extreme care, as wound healing problems are serious. The paratenon is identified and incised. In patients with evidence of coexisting paratendinopathy, the scarred and thickened tissue is generally excised. The tendon is incised sharply in line with the tendon fibers bundles. The tendinopathic tissue can be identified as it generally has lost its shiny appearance, and it frequently contains disorganized fiber bundles that have more of a “crabmeat” appearance (Fig. 10.7). This tissue is sharply excised. The remaining gap can be repaired using a side-to-side repair, but we leave it unsutured. If significant loss of tendon tissue occurs during the débridement, a tendon augmentation or transfer should be consider, even if we rarely undertake this additional procedure. The subcutaneous tissues are sutured with absorbable material; the skin edges are juxtaposed with Steri-Strips and a routine compressive bandage. The limb is immobilized in a below-knee weight-bearing cast with the foot plantigrade. A period of initial splinting and crutch walking allows pain and swelling to subside after surgery. After 14 days, the wound is inspected, and motion exercises are initiated. The patient is encouraged to start daily active and passive ankle range-of-motion exercises. The use of a removable walker boot can be helpful during this phase. Early weight bearing after uncomplicated procedures is encouraged. However, extensive débridements and tendon transfers may require protected weight bearing for 4–6 weeks postoperatively. After 6–8 weeks, more intensive strengthening exercises are started, gradually progressing to plyometrics and eventually running and jumping.

A systematic review of the literature showed successful results in over 70 % of cases [68], but these relatively high success rates are not always observed in clinical practice, probably because of the poor methods scores of many articles. Patients should be informed of the potential failure of the procedure, risk of wound complications, and at times prolonged recovery time. Possible complications of this surgical procedure are wound breakdown (3 %), sural nerve injury (1 %), superficial or deep infection (2.5 %), and deep vein thrombosis [69]. Achilles tendon rupture has been reported after surgery for tendinopathy in a patient performing eccentric loading exercises.

10.8 Synthesis and Therapeutic Indications

Achilles tendinopathy is a common cause of disability both in athletic and sedentary population. The etiopathogenesis is currently considered multifactorial, but precise pathogenetic mechanisms are still largely unclear.

Even though there is a consensus on the importance of preventive exercises programs and different protocols have been proposed, the evidence on their long-term effectiveness is little. Eccentric exercises are realistically effective to manage AT in up to two-thirds of patients.

There is some evidence for benefit for high-energy ESWT in midportion AT. However, conservative management is unsuccessful in 24–45.5 % of patients, and surgery is recommended after 6 months of conservative management. Long-standing AT is associated with poor postoperative results, with a greater rate of reoperation before reaching an acceptable outcome.

Both minimally invasive and open surgical techniques have been described. Good results have been reported with minimally invasive techniques, even though well-conducted level I evidence studies are lacking. They offer many advantages like reduced local morbidity and risks of infection, they are technically easy to perform and relatively inexpensive, and they can be associated with conservative treatment or other minimally invasive procedures to optimize the results.

References

1. Vora AM, Myerson MS, Oliva F, Mafulli N (2005) Tendinopathy of the main body of the Achilles tendon. Foot Ankle Clin 10:293–308
2. Maffulli N, Sharma P, Luscombe KL (2004) Achilles tendinopathy: aetiology and management. J R Soc Med 97:472–476
3. Rolf CMT (1997) Etiology, histopathology, and outcome of surgery in achillodynia. Foot Ankle Int 18:565–569
4. Rompe JD, Furia JP, Maffulli N (2008) Mid-portion Achilles tendinopathy: current options for treatment. Disabil Rehabil 30:1666–1676
5. Astrom M (1998) Partial rupture in Achilles tendinopathy. A retrospective analysis of 342 cases. Acta Orthop Scand 69:404–407
6. Ronga M, Oliva F, Vigneti D et al (2009) Achilles tendinopathy. Physiopathology. In: Maffulli N, Oliva F (eds) Achilles tendon. CIC Edizioni internazionali, Rome, pp 39–45
7. Nigg B (1994) The role of impact forces and foot pronation: a new paradigm. Clin J Sports Med 11:2–9
8. Bryant AL, Clark RA, Bartold S et al (2008) Effects of oestrogen on the mechanical behavior of the human Achilles tendon in vivo. J Appl Physiol 105:1035–1043
9. Circi E, Akpinar S, Akgun RC et al (2009) Biomechanical and histological comparison of the influence of oestrogen deficient state on tendon healing potential in rats. Int Orthop 33:1461–1466
10. Cook JL, Bass SL, Black JE (2007) Hormone therapy is associated with smaller Achilles tendon diameter in active postmenopausal women. Scand J Med Sci Sports 17:128–132
11. Torricelli P, Veronesi F, Pagani S et al (2013) In vitro tenocyte metabolism in aging and oestrogen deficiency. Age (Dordr) 35:2125–2136

12. Ahmed N (2005) Advanced glycation endproducts – role in pathology of diabetic complications. Diabetes Res Clin Pract 67:3–21
13. Gautieri A, Redaelli A, Buehler MJ et al (2014) Age- and diabetes-related nonenzymatic cross-links in collagen fibrils: candidate amino acids involved in advanced glycation endproducts. Matrix Biol 34:89–95
14. Li Y, Fessel G, Georgiadis M et al (2013) Advanced glycation end-products diminish tendon collagen fiber sliding. Matrix Biol 32:169–177
15. Duncan WS (1928) The relationship of hyperthysoidism to joint conditions. J Am Med Assoc 91:1779
16. Oliva F, Berardi AC, Misiti S, Verza Felzacappa C, Iacone A, Maffulli N (2013) Thyroid hormones enhance growth and counteract apoptosis in human tenocytes isolated from rotator cuff tendons. Cell Death Dis 4:e705
17. Berardi A, Oliva F, Berardocco M, La Rovere M, Accorsi P, Maffulli N (2014) Thyroid hormones increase collagen I and cartilage matrix protein (COMP) expression in vitro human tenocytes. Muscles Ligaments Tendons J 4:285–291
18. Warrender WJ, Brown OL, Abboud JA (2011) Outcomes of arthroscopic rotator cuff repairs in obese patients. J Shoulder Elbow Surg 20:961–967
19. Giai Via A, De Cupis M, Spoliti M et al (2013) Clinical and biological aspects of rotator cuff tears. Muscles Ligaments Tendons J 3:70–92
20. Gaida JE, Cook JL, Bass SL (2008) Adiposity and tendinopathy. Disabil Rehabil 30:1555–1562
21. Abate M, Oliva F, Schiavone C et al (2012) Achilles tendinopathy in amateur runners role of adiposity (tendinopathies and obesity). Muscles Ligaments Tendons J 2:44–48
22. Biancalana A, Veloso LA, Gomes L (2010) Obesity affects collagen fibril diameter and mechanical properties of tendons in Zucker rats. Connect Tissue Res 51:171–178
23. Hills AP, Hennig EM, Byrne NM et al (2006) The biomechanics of adiposity – structural and functional limitations of obesity and implications for movement. Obes Rev 7:13–24
24. Waggett AD, Ralphs JR, Kwan AP et al (1998) Characterization of collagens and proteoglycans at the insertion of the human Achilles tendon. Matrix Biol 16:457–470
25. Modesti A, Oliva F (2013) All is around ECM of tendons?! Muscles Ligaments Tendons J 3:1
26. Dalton S, Cawston TE, Riley GP, Bayley IJ, Hazleman BL (1995) Human shoulder tendon biopsy samples in organ culture produce procollagenase and tissue inhibitor of metalloproteinases. Ann Rheum Dis 54:571–577
27. Choi HR, Kondo S, Hirose K et al (2002) Expression and enzymatic activity of MMP-2 during healing process of the acute suprasupinatus tendon tear in rabbits. J Orthop Res 20:927–933
28. Riley GP, Curry V, DeGroot J et al (2002) Matrix metalloproteinase activities and their relationship with collagen remodelling in tendon pathology. Matrix Biol 21:185–195
29. Tarantino U, Oliva F, Taurisano G et al (2009) FXIIIA and TGF-beta over-expression produces normal musculoskeletal phenotype in TG2–/–mice. Amino Acids 36:679–684
30. Oliva F, Zocchi L, Codispoti A et al (2009) Transglutaminases expression in human supraspinatus tendon ruptures and in mouse tendons. Biochem Biophys Res Commun 20:887–891
31. Dean BJ, Franklin SL, Carr AJ (2013) The peripheral neuronal phenotype is important in the pathogenesis of painful human tendinopathy: a systematic review. Clin Orthop Relat Res 471:3036–3046
32. Andres KH, von During M, Schmidt RF (1985) Sensory innervation of the Achilles tendon by group III and IV afferent fibers. Anat Embryol (Berl) 172:145–156
33. van Sterkenburg M, van Dijk N (2011) Mid-portion Achilles tendinopathy: why painful? An evidence-based philosophy. Knee Surg Sports Traumatol Arthrosc 19:1367–1375
34. Alfredson H, Ohberg L, Forsgren S (2003) Is vasculo-neural ingrowth the cause of pain in chronic Achilles tendinosis? An investigation using ultrasonography and colour Doppler, immunohistochemistry, and diagnostic injections. Knee Surg Sports Traumatol Arthrosc 11:334–338
35. Schizas N, Weiss R, Lian O, Frihagen F, Bahr R, Ackermann PW (2012) Glutamate receptors in tendinopathic patients. J Orthop Res 30:1447–1452

36. Steyaert AE, Burssens PJ, Vercruysse CW, Vanderstraeten GG, Verbeeck RM (2006) The effects of substance P on the biomechanic properties of ruptured rat Achilles' tendon. Arch Phys Med Rehabil 87:254–258
37. Rogers BS, Leach RE (1996) Achilles tendinitis. Foot Ankle Clin 1:249–259
38. Binfield PM, Maffulli N (1997) Surgical management of common tendinopathies of the lower limb. Sports Exerc Injury 3:116–122
39. Maffulli N, Testa V, Capasso G et al (2006) Surgery for chronic Achilles tendinopathy yields worse results in nonathletic patients. Clin J Sport Med 16:123–128
40. Maffulli N, Wong J, Almekinders LC (2003) Types and epidemiology of tendinopathy. Clin Sports Med 22:675–692
41. Rompe JD, Nafe B, Furia JP et al (2007) Eccentric loading, shock-wave treatment, or a wait-and-see policy for tendinopathy of the main body of tendon Achilles: a randomized controlled trial. Am J Sports Med 35:374–383
42. Petersa JA, Zwervera J, Diercksa RL, Elferink-Gemserb MT, van den Akker-Scheeka I (2016) Preventive interventions for tendinopathy: a systematic review. J Sci Med Sport 19:205–211
43. Pope R, Herbert R, Kirwan J (1998) Effects of ankle dorsiflexion range and pre-exercise calf muscle stretching on injury risk in Army recruits. Aust J Physiother 44:165–172
44. Amako M, Oda T, Masuoka K et al (2003) Effect of static stretching on prevention of injuries for military recruits. Mil Med 168:442–446
45. Kraemer R, Knobloch K (2009) A soccer-specific balance training program for ham-string muscle and patellar and achilles tendon injuries: an intervention study in premier league female soccer. Am J Sports Med 37:1384–1393.26
46. House C, Reece A, Roiz de Sa D (2013) Shock-absorbing insoles reduce the incidence of lower limb overuse injuries sustained during Royal Marine training. Mil Med 178:683–689
47. Milgrom C, Finestone A, Shlamkovitch N, Wosk J, Laor A, Voloshin A et al (1992) Prevention of overuse injuries of the foot by improved shoe shock attenuation. A randomized prospective study. Clin Orthop Relat Res (281):189–192
48. Larsen K, Weidich F, Leboeuf-Yde C (2002) Can custom-made biomechanic shoe orthoses prevent problems in the back and lower extremities? A randomized, controlled intervention trial of 146 military conscripts. J Manipulative Physiol Ther 25:326–331
49. Longo UG, Ronga M, Maffulli N (2009) Achilles tendinopathy. Sports Med Arthrosc 17(2):112–126
50. Stanish WD, Rubinovich RM, Curwin S (2008) Eccentric exercise in chronic tendinitis. Clin Orthop Relat Res 1986:65–68
51. Fahlstrom M, Jonsson P, Lorentzon R et al (2003) Chronic Achilles tendon pain treated with eccentric calf-muscle training. Knee Surg Sports Traumatol Arthrosc 11:327–333
52. Norregaard J, Larsen CC, Bieler T et al (2007) Eccentric exercise in treatment of Achilles tendinopathy. Scand J Med Sci Sports 17:133–138
53. Alfredson H, Pietila T, Jonsson P et al (1998) Heavy-load eccentric calf muscle training for the treatment of chronic Achilles tendinosis. Am J Sports Med 26:360–366
54. Roos E, Engstrom M, Lagerquist A et al (2004) Clinical improvement after 6 weeks of eccentric exercise in patients with mid-portion Achilles tendinopathy – a randomized trial with 1-year follow-up. Scand J Med Sci Sports 14:286–295
55. de Vos RJ, Weir A, Visser RJ et al (2007) The additional value of a night splint to eccentric exercises in chronic midportion Achilles tendinopathy: a randomised controlled trial. Br J Sports Med 41:e5
56. Sayana MK, Maffulli N (2007) Eccentric calf muscle training in non-athletic patients with Achilles tendinopathy. J Sci Med Sport 10:52–58
57. Lohrer H, Scholl J, Arentz S (2002) Achilles tendinopathy and patellar tendinopathy. Results of radial shockwave therapy in patients with unsuccessfully treated tendinoses. Sportverletz Sportschaden 16:108–114
58. Peers K (2003) Extracorporeal shock wave therapy in chronic Achilles and patellar tendinopathy. Leuven University Press, Leuven, pp 61–75

59. Speed C (2014) A systematic review of shockwave therapies in soft tissue conditions: focusing on the evidence. Br J Sports Med 48:1538–1542
60. Costa ML, Shepstone L, Donell ST et al (2005) Shock wave therapy for chronic Achilles tendon pain: a randomized placebo-controlled trial. Clin Orthop Relat Res 440:199–204
61. Rasmussen S, Christensen M, Mathiesen I et al (2008) Shockwave therapy for chronic Achilles tendinopathy: a double-blind, randomized clinical trial of efficacy. Acta Orthop 79:249–256
62. Loppini M, Maffulli N (2012) Conservative management of tendinopathy: an evidence-based approach. Muscles Ligaments Tendons J 1:134–137
63. Chan O, O'Dowd D, Padhiar N et al (2008) High volume image guided injections in chronic Achilles tendinopathy. Disabil Rehabil 30:1697–1708
64. Maffulli N, Spiezia F, Longo UG, Denaro V, Maffulli GD (2013) High volume image guided injections for the management of chronic tendinopathy of the main body of the Achilles tendon. Phys Ther Sport 14:163–167
65. de Vos RJ, Weir A, van Schie HT et al (2010) Platelet-rich plasma injection for chronic Achilles tendinopathy: a randomized controlled trial. JAMA 303:144–149
66. Testa V, Capasso G, Benazzo F, Maffulli N (2002) Management of Achilles tendinopathy by ultrasound-guided percutaneous tenotomy. Med Sci Sports Exerc 34:573–580
67. Maffulli N, Testa V, Capasso G, Bifulco G, Binfield PM (1997) Results of percutaneous longitudinal tenotomy for Achilles tendinopathy in middle- and long-distance runners. Am J Sports Med 25:835–840
68. Tallon C, Coleman BD, Khan KM, Maffuli N (2001) Outcome of surgery for chronic Achilles tendinopathy: a critical review. Am J Sports Med 29:315–320
69. Paavola M, Orava S, Leppilahti J, Kannus P, Jarvinen M (2000) Chronic achilles tendon overuse injury: complications after surgical treatment: an analysis of 432 consecutive patients. Am J Sports Med 28:77–82

Chapter 11
Patellar Tendinopathy

Piero Volpi, E. Prospero, C. Bait, G. Carimati, V.P. Di Francia, P. Felisaz, and L. Balzarini

Abstract Patellar tendon tendinopathies have always been an important and recurring issue in many sports. Even in the case of the patellar tendon, the first hypothesis of inflammatory pathogenesis has been replaced by the degenerative theory, and the term "tendinitis" was soon replaced with that of "tendinopathy." In addition to the hypothesis inflammatory, over the years, several theories have been formulated in the context of its pathogenesis. Conservative treatment proposed by various authors and that is possible to find retrievable in the literature ranges from functional rest, the use of nonsteroidal anti-inflammatory drugs, modification of training techniques, stretching, and eccentric training. However, a not insignificant number of athletes demonstrate nonresponsiveness in respect of conservative therapies, and in front of a long period of persistence of symptoms, a surgical solution must be considered.

11.1 Introduction

Patellar tendinopathy is a common overuse condition of the patellar tendon and represents an important problem for athletes of different sports.

It most commonly affects jumping athletes from young age to adulthood, and it is an acute/chronic injury of patellar tendon.

P. Volpi (✉)
Humanitas Clinical Institute, IRCCS, Rozzano, Milan, Italy

FC Internazionale Medical Staff, Milano, Italy
e-mail: volpi.piero@libero.it

E. Prospero • C. Bait • G. Carimati • V.P. Di Francia • P. Felisaz • L. Balzarini
Humanitas Clinical Institute, IRCCS, Rozzano, Milan, Italy

G.N. Bisciotti, P. Volpi (eds.), *The Lower Limb Tendinopathies*, Sports and Traumatology, DOI 10.1007/978-3-319-33234-5_11

Basketball and volleyball are the sports more interested by these pathologies, respectively, with an incidence of 31.9 and 44.6 % [1] mostly because of the mechanics of sport-specific gestures, characterized by high-speed and power demand on the extensor apparatus. This disease was described in 1973 by Blazina as "jumper's knee" and this definition has been preserved until now [2].

Clinically it is characterized by an anterior pain load-dependent at the inferior pole of the patella, to the tendon or at distal insertion of it.

The majority of cases resolve with nonsurgical treatment; rest, cryotherapy, eccentric exercise, extracorporeal shockwave therapy, magnetic fields, and PRP therapy are the most commonly used.

Patellar tendinopathy implies a difficult management by the athlete because of the severe symptomatology and severe impairment of sports performance or because of the long period of stop; more then half of the athletes still have some symptoms after their carrier ended [3–5]

Chronically stressed tendons, at the last stage of the degenerative process, can end in tendon rupture.

In this chapter, we will discuss about the pathology, clinical and instrumental diagnosis, and therapeutic approach.

11.2 Epidemiology and Etiopathogenesis

Patellar tendinopathy is very common among athletes and nonathletes [6].

Mainly it involves people who repeat flexion extension movement under load or, as cited above, sports player with an incidence of up to 40 % in certain sports; an important role is played by overload and reduced loading capacity by the athletes.

Prevalence of patellar tendinopathy ranges from 5 to 45 % in sports players [7–9] with an incidence peak between 15 and 30 years – it is the period in which most patients practice sport activities.

Prevalence is higher in males and affected persons usually are between 15 and 40 years.

Different risk factors for the diseases are described and can be classified as intrinsic and extrinsic.

Intrinsic risk factors cannot be modified and can give information about which groups have to be monitored:

- Gender: the incidence is higher in male than females. This was due to different capacity in generating force and to the ability of the athletic movement [1]. Estrogens may have a protective role on the tendons [10].
- Age: the tendinopathy is considered to be linked to overload, so the greater the age the greater the stress on the tendon at the same level of sport activity.
- Rheumatologic diseases and collagenopathies: they can change the structure of the tendon and decrease the mechanical resistance.

- Injury of the contralateral tendon: patients with a contralateral overload can be more susceptible for developing pathologies of the other tendon.
- Anatomy: there are different opinions about anatomical features predisposing to jumper's knee tendinopathy [11].

Extrinsic risk factors are the most interesting for the professional sportsman and are the once for whom it's possible to apply preventive measures.

- Environment and playground: in volleyball and basketball players, it was shown that a harder ground increases the risk of developing the tendinopathy [1]. In recreational players, no differences were indicated between the incidence of the pathology in athletes playing on natural ground and the incidence in athletes playing on synthetic ground.
- Sport-specific gestures: it is impossible to modify them but it is possible to improve the technique of execution to reduce the load and the frequency of execution in at risk or symptomatic people.
- Equipments: mechanical properties of footwear can change the friction coefficient and the mechanical load on the limb. It is important to choose the best footwear according to the features of the ground, in order to reduce microtrauma from impact with the ground. More often knee bandages are used to reduce the load on the tendon in athletes who have early symptoms, but their benefit is doubtful.
- Exposition level: many hours of training and sport are the most important risk factors for the development of patellar tendon pathology [3, 12]. Some authors have shown a relation between the risk of developing the jumper's knee and 12 h/week training; the same link has been pointed out with 5 h/week training with weights [13, 14]. This is the risk factor more difficult to manage.

11.3 Anatomy and Biomechanics

Patellar tendon is an anatomical structure interposed between the height of patella and the tibial anterior apophysis; the main elements of tendon are collagen, cells, and extracellular matrix. The main task of the collagen is to provide the tensile strength, while tenocytes produce extracellular matrix and procollagen [15].

It is the terminal part of the thigh's extensor apparatus responsible for leg extension, so the tendon supports the work of the muscles and endures a high mechanical stress, mostly at the level of its patellar origin and its tibial insertion. The extensor apparatus can perform both eccentric and concentric work. Patellar tendon is very durable to tensile force and it is proven that a very high strength is required to break a healthy tendon [16, 17]. However, the continuous stress, due to repetitive sport-specific gestures, can lead to an overload pathology.

There are other theories about the pathogenesis of patellar tendinopathy, as mechanical, vascular, or nervous causes [18, 19].

Patellar tendon is stressed in different ways according to the degree of knee flexion: between 45° and 60°, the position of the patellae and the high forces exerted on the tendon result in a higher probability of having injuries, above during eccentric work [20]. The greatest muscle strength, produced in an eccentric way, is 1.5–2 times higher than the greatest isometric force and the higher concentric force, above at high speeds [21]. The force transmitted from the ground varies according to different athletic feats and corresponds to 2.8 times the body weight during long-distance running, to 6 times the body weight during volleyball jumping, and to 10 times the body weight during the takeoff of the long jump [22]. The highest forces of load transmission to the quadriceps occur during the ballistic reaction with the "drop jumps," during which the forces transmitted to the quadriceps are proportional to the reaction force of the ground. So it is reasonable to assume a link between the working model of the quadriceps and the prevalence of the jumper's knee. This assumption seems to be validated by the distribution of the prevalence reported in several studies. This is highest in basketball, volleyball, and athletics and low or negligible in other sports.

11.4 Pathogenesis

The etiology of tendinopathy is not clear and generally has a multifactorial origin; tendinopathy is usually the result of tendon nonhealing and often the affected tendon shows no sign of inflammation but, on the contrary, shows increased new blood vessels, fibroblasts, hypercellularity, and disorganized collagen [23].

Histopathological studies concerning patellar tendinopathy show the separation of the collagen fibers with eventual loss of the normal organization, a most fundamental mucoid substance, morphological changes of tenocytes, fibrocartilaginous metaplasia, and cellular and capillary proliferation [24, 25].

The connection between the conditions of mechanical load and the pathophysiological response is unknown. It was suggested that the mechanical overload can produce partial ruptures in the tendon tissue and the histological results have been interpreted as partial tendon ruptures [8, 9, 14]. The hypoechoic lesions, observed in the proximal patellar tendon, associated to tendinopathy are usually described as a result of the failed healing or as partial tendon ruptures.

Some classical theories suppose that the lack of traction promotes healing and adaptation of tension; a too high traction might prevent healing and promote the accumulation of degenerative tissue. Other authors suggest that an excessive mechanical stretching of the tenocytes may activate some signal pathways able to induce apoptosis. Histological findings, observed during tendinopathy, are compatible with an apoptotic process. It can be possible that, when the mechanical load is higher than the adaptive response of tenocytes, apoptosis is induced [26].

Pain, in tendinopathy, in the past was attributed to inflammation, but new studies and new theories have shown that pain originates from biochemical and mechanical factors [15].

Rupture of the patellar tendon is considered by many authors as the final event of the degenerative disease. These injuries usually occur in more than 40-year-old people and often are associated with metabolic or systemic disease and just occasionally may be bilateral.

11.5 Clinical Examination

Patellar tendinopathy is characterized by pain; it can manifest in an acute, subacute, or in an intermittent way, usually not following local trauma; it can be associated to a change in the type or in the frequency of training, to a work overload. Usually the pain is reported in specific sites, mostly located at the level of insertion near the lower apex of the patella (Fig. 11.1); in the remaining cases, the pain can be localized to the tendon or to the distal insertion of it. For a long time, the clinical classification more commonly followed was the Blazina's one that was improved and divided into six stages according to clinical symptoms (Table 11.1).

In the first Blazina's classification, the last step was related to the catastrophic rupture of the patellar tendon, a rare but possible eventuality. Usually the symptoms described above disappear with a break from sports activities, especially if it is the

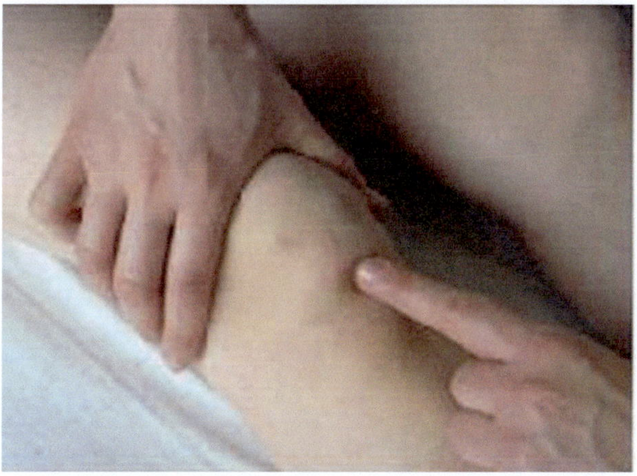

Fig. 11.1 Pain in lower apex of patella

Table 11.1 Classification of patellar tendinopathy according to clinical symptoms

Stage 0	No pain
Stage I	Rare pain with normal performance
Stage II	Moderate pain during sports activities with normal performance
Stage III	Pain during sports activities with initial qualitative or quantitative limitation of performance
Stage IV	Pain during sports activities with an important decrement of performance
Stage V	Pain during daily life and impossibility in practice sport

first episode, but symptoms can recur if the patient resumes physical training too early or with excessive workloads. More attention should be paid to the recovery time of patients with chronic tendinopathy. Concerning patellar tendon rupture, the physician should carefully evaluate the swelling and the hematoma in the patella that can be associated with a hemarthrosis. The more evident and limiting clinical sign is the inability to an active extension of the leg and to lift the extended limb; this makes the gait difficult also using some aids.

11.6 Instrumental Diagnosis

Patellar tendon injuries can be investigated with conventional radiography, ultrasonography, and MRI.

Standard radiograph could be useful in detecting indirect sign of tendon injuries and may detect abnormalities such as cortex irregularities at the lower pole of the patella or at tibial tuberosity, with insertional or peritendinous calcifications and in case of traumatic cortical sleeve fractures.

Fragmented ossification centers in the Osgood-Schlatter or Sinding-Larsen-Johansson diseases and bipartite patella are common radiological direct sign of pathology.

In the case of patellar tendon rupture, knee radiographs with lateral projections may display proximal dislocation of the patella (high patella or high riding patella) and bone avulsions (Fig. 11.2)

Ultrasonography with linear high-resolution probes allows proper visualization of the tendon structure with high resolution.

It may detect loss of the fibrillar architecture and the presence of intratendinous hypoechoic areas, associated with perilesional edema variably extended.

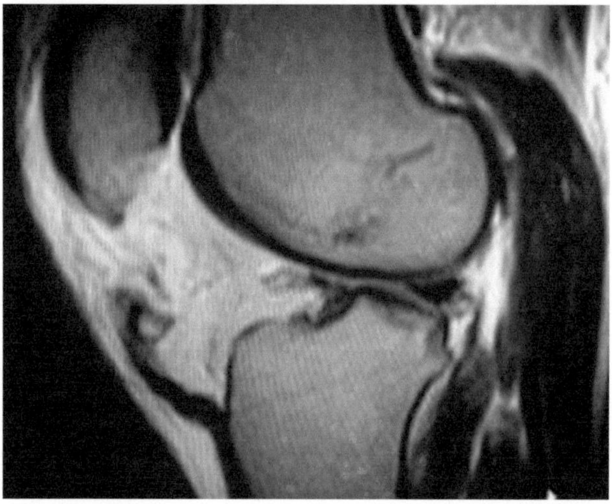

Fig. 11.2 Bone avulsion

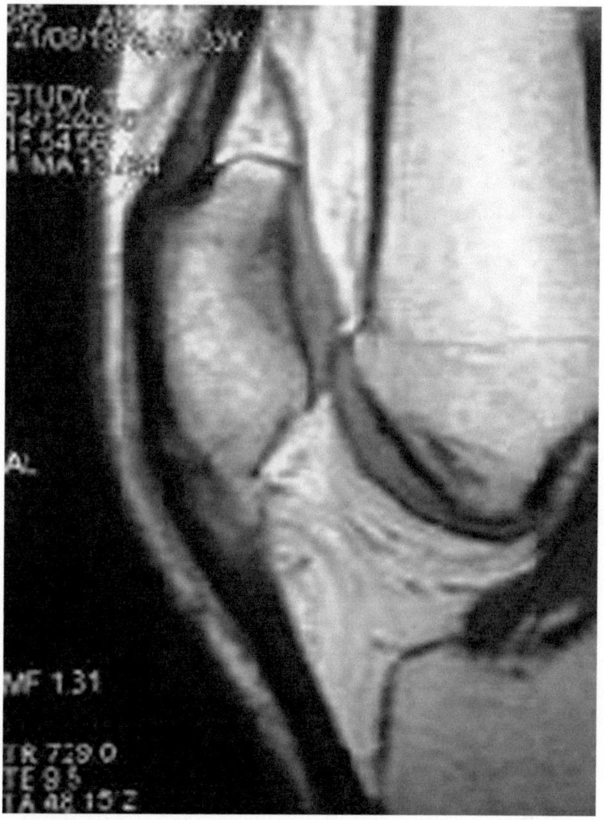

Fig. 11.3 Proximal patellar tendinopathy

Ultrasound is suitable also in patients with patellar fractures, for assessing the hemorrhage, the involvement of the surrounding soft tissues, and the integrity of the patellar tendon.

Ultrasound is a low-cost and safe technique that may be repeated regularly in the follow-up of a patellar tendon injury.

Furthermore, it is limited by the small field of view and inter-operator variability, and hence skilled operators are required. MRI is the most accurate and safe examination for assessing directly patellar tendon pathology, with best demonstration of the morphology (site and extension of fibers solution).

A regular tendon should appear with very low signal in all sequences.

Areas of intratendinous high signal intensity on T1-weighted images depend on tendon degeneration (Fig. 11.3), while hyperintensity in T2-weighted images is referred to edema or hemorrhage.

A common pitfall in patellar tendon MR imaging is the "magic angle effect," a hyperintensity artifact only seen with short TE (time of echo) sequences such as T1W that disappears with long echo time in T2W images [27].

Thickening and deformation of proximal patellar tendon are associated with chronic tendonitis [28, 29].

Swelling of the Hoffa's fat pad and the regional bursae may be present in long-standing tendinopathy or severe tendon injuries.

Bone edema at the enthesis is also a common indirect sign in case of acute-subacute enthesopathy but conspicuous edema may conceal a patellar/tibial sleeve fracture.

So MRI should be done in patients elected for surgical repair to evaluate direct tendon and associated capsular, ligamentous, or meniscal injuries.

11.7 Treatment

Usually the treatment for a sports player affected by patellar tendinopathy is conservative; surgery is often postponed. The treatment should be carefully planned and the physician should modulate and quantify the type, the load and the timing of exercise, the abstention from particular activities, and the rest period. The athlete needs to be informed about what happened and a protocol should be started for the reeducation, rehabilitation, and redistribution of the load and of the intensity of work. The sportsman, during the symptomatic period, should begin a training including all kind of exercises but mostly eccentric ones and stretching. These are suggested to all patients with acute tendinopathy, working mainly on the phase of deceleration and on gradual recovery of elasticity; this treatment can be associated with hydrokinesitherapy and with manual massage to relax quadriceps.

Most important are the modulation and the type of physical activity; if the patient is unable to participate in a usual activity, he or she must find an alternative fitness activity. The patient must promote eccentric exercises. We can divide therapies medically and physically. The medical ones help to solve the clinical symptoms; for this reason, there are many drugs available, above NSAIDs, with systemic and local action. It is important to remember that prolonged use of NSAIDs may have negative effects on long-term tendon healing [30]. There are different opinions about appropriateness of local injections of steroidal anti-inflammatory drugs (SAIDs); these can be useful in reducing symptoms temporarily, but on the other hand these can cause tendon ruptures. In order to improve the clinical symptoms, physical therapies can be performed. Cryotherapy, tens, laser, ultrasound, tecartherapy, shockwave, and magnetic fields are the most used techniques on the tendon to relieve pain. Especially the shockwave seems to play an additional role in stimulating tendon tissue regeneration [31, 32]. Another kind of therapy that has spread in the last decade for the patellar tendinopathy is the injection with autologous platelet-rich plasma (PRP) [33] with the purpose to stimulate healing of the tendon tissue using platelet growth factors. One or more injections can be performed in a few days. Comparing them with shockwave seems that the results of PRP injections are better

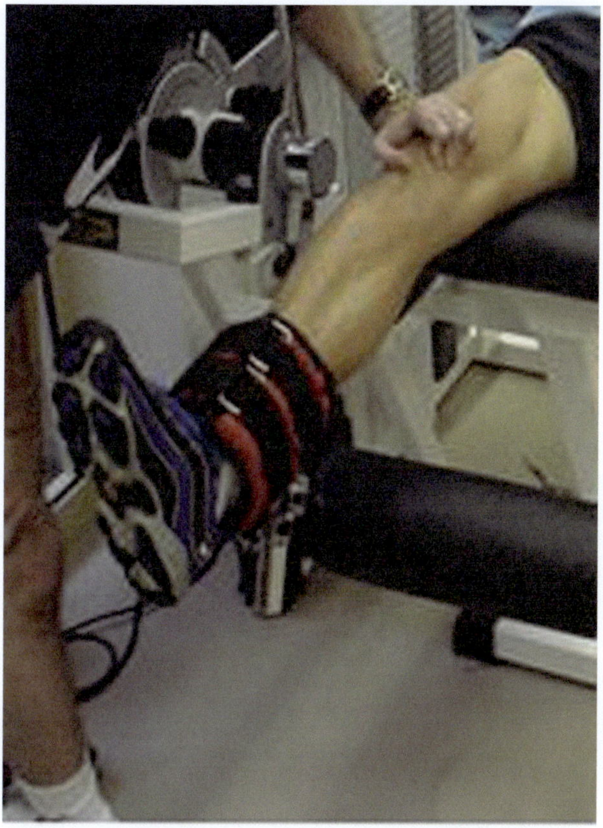

Fig. 11.4 Eccentric exercise

from the biological point of view [34]. Anyway in the literature, the results are controversial, mostly because of the different method of preparation and concentration of the substance to inject [35].

With regard to physical therapy, the most used exercise for the treatment of tendinopathy is based on eccentric work (Fig. 11.4). During those exercises, a lengthening of the muscle-tendon unit with the load with a repetitive loading and unloading in the tendon is observed; this seems to have an important role for the tropism of the tendon and for the reduction of pain [36, 37].

This approach in patients affected by patellar tendinopathy might allow the recovery of the sport activities in a period ranging from a few weeks up to 6 months; if symptoms persists or worsen, surgery should be considered. There are various surgical options but all have as their main purpose, the stimulation and facilitation of the tendon healing. Since in most cases the tendinopathy is proximal, the most used surgical approach consists of some steps: slice longitudinally the tendon for a

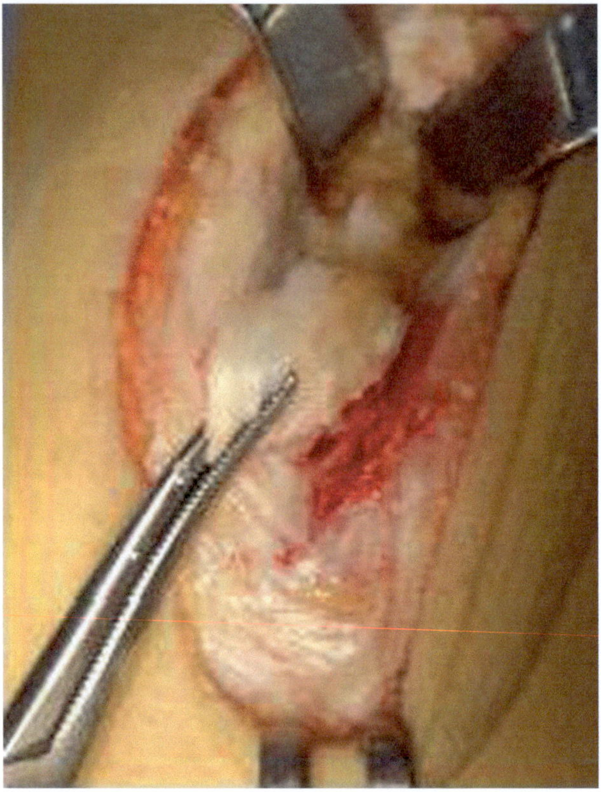

Fig. 11.5 Degenerated tissue removal

few centimeters, in correspondence with the injured area, previously evaluated with MRI; remove the part of possible degenerated tendon tissue (Fig. 11.5); and perform a cruentation of the patellar apex and some small perforations in the apex in order to facilitate the flow of blood in the interested area. It is possible to perform some tendon scarification if the injured area is extended. The same procedure can be used in case of distal tendinopathy, performing scarifications and perforations of the ATA, eventually associated with the removal of the degenerated tissue. During the execution of this surgical technique, it is possible to use PRP gel (Fig. 11.6).

In case of patellar tendon rupture (Fig. 11.7), a discriminating factor able to condition a good outcome of the surgical treatment and of the function recovery is the time since the accident. The injuries treated in the acute phase seem to have a better complete functional recovery. The surgical treatment of the acute rupture of the proximal or distal insertion of the patellar tendon consists in the reinsertion of the tendon to the bone component. It can be made using or transosseous sutures or suture anchors in order to restore the bone-tendon continuity. This first step has to be associated to a biological augmentation (Fig. 11.8) in reabsorbable or not

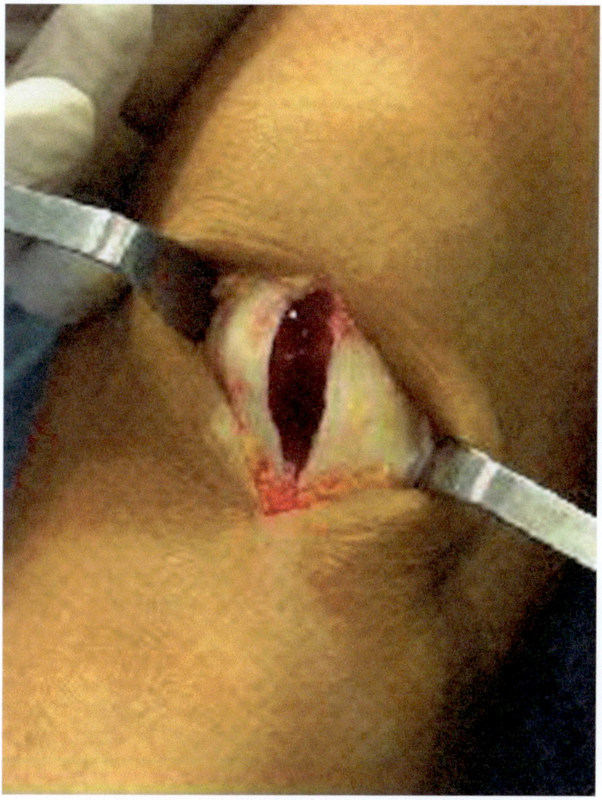

Fig. 11.6 PRP

reabsorbable material [20]. Some author suggests also a transosseous wire augmentation.

In case of ruptures of the central part of the tendon, the continuity of it have to be restored taking back the patella to its original site and eventually associating an augmentation, biological or in reabsorbable material. Also in this case, there are authors who suggest a transosseous wire augmentation. Often if lesions are unrecognized or chronic, perilesional or calcific scar tissue is present associated to anatomical deformity of knee detectable at the physical examination. In this case, the surgical approach is more complex with the possible difficulty to recover the right position of the patella. The treatment consists in the initial removal of the scar tissue and calcifications and in the cruentation of the ends of tendon. Sometimes the gap cannot be filled without a "zed" elongation of the patellar tendon. If the ruptures are inveterate with a considerable ascent of the patella, it is possible to use the technique suggested by Dejour, transplanting the distal part of the extensor apparatus of the contralateral knee [38]. Alternatively tendon allograft or autologous tendon transplantation (semitendinosus and gracilis tendons) can be used to minimize the iatrogenic lesions for the contralateral healthy knee.

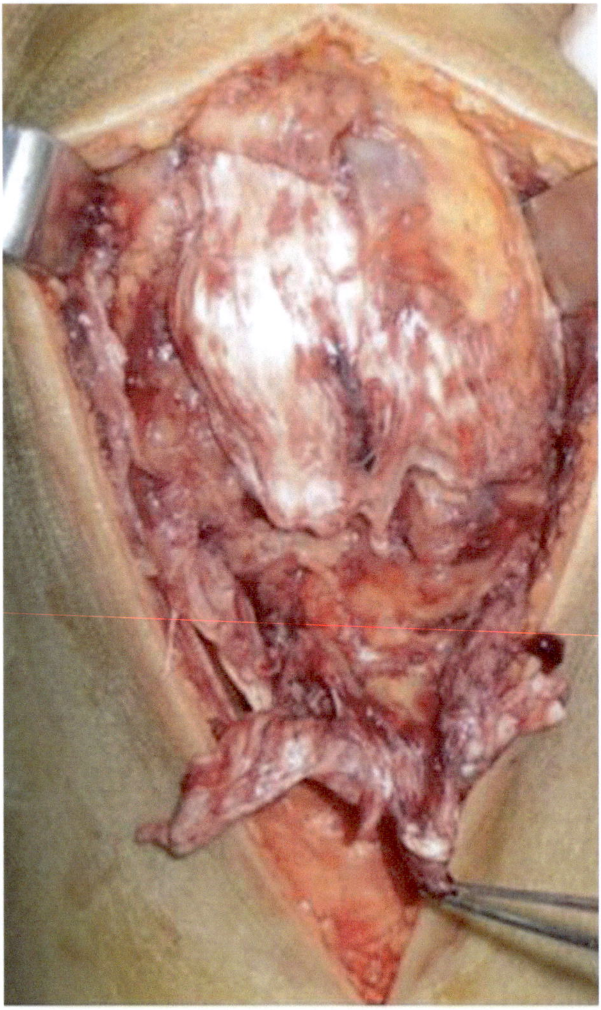

Fig. 11.7 Patellar tendon rupture

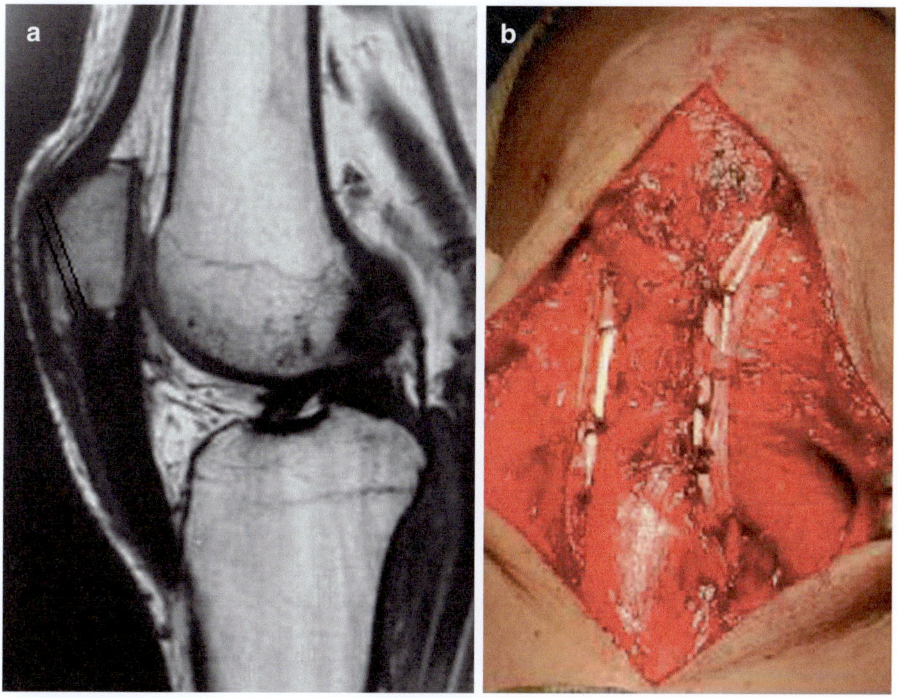

Fig. 11.8 (**a**) Transosseous suture; (**b**) biological augmentation

Bibliography

1. Lian OB, Engebretsen L, Bahr R (2005) Prevalence of jumper's knee among elite athletes from different sports: a cross-sectional study. Am J Sports Med 33(4):561–567, Epub 2005 Feb 8
2. Blazina ME, Kerlan RK, Jobe FW, Carter VS, Carlson GJ (1973) Jumper's knee. Orthop Clin North Am 4(3):665–678
3. Hägglund M, Zwerver J, Ekstrand J (2011) Epidemiology of patellar tendinopathy in elite male soccer players. Am J Sports Med 39(9):1906–1911, Epub 2011 Jun 3
4. Ferretti A (1986) Epidemiology of jumper's knee. Sports Med 3(4):289–295
5. Fredberg U, Bolvig L, Andersen NT (2008) Prophylactic training in asymptomatic soccer players with ultrasonographic abnormalities in Achilles and patellar tendons: the Danish Super League Study. Am J Sports Med 36(3):451–460, Epub 2007 Dec 13
6. Stanish WD, Rubinovich RM, Curwin S (1986) Eccentric exercise in chronic tendinitis. Clin Orthop Relat Res. (208):65–68
7. Raatikainen T, Karpakka J, Puranen J, Orava S (1994) Operative treatment of partial rupture of the patellar ligament. A study of 138 cases. Int J Sports Med 15(1):46–49
8. Martens M, Wouters P, Burssens A, Mulier JC (1982) Patellar tendinitis: pathology and results of treatment. Acta Orthop Scand 53(3):445–450
9. Karlsson J, Lundin O, Lossing IW, Peterson L (1991) Partial rupture of the patellar ligament. Results after operative treatment. Am J Sports Med 19(4):403–408

10. Cook JL, Bass SL, Black JE (2007) Hormone therapy is associated with smaller Achilles tendon diameter in active post-menopausal women. Scand J Med Sci Sports 17:128–132
11. Khan KM, Cook JL, Maffulli N (2005) Patellar Tendinopathy and Patellar Tendon Rupture. Tendon injuries. In: Maffulli N, Renström P, Leadbetter WB (eds). Springer Edition, Switzerland
12. Gaida JE, Cook JL, Bass SL, Austen S, Kiss ZS (2004) Are unilateral and bilateral patellar tendinopathy distinguished by differences in anthropometry, body composition, or muscle strength in elite female basketball players? Br J Sports Med 38(5):581–585
13. Cook JL, Khan KM, Kiss ZS, Griffiths L (2000) Patellar tendinopathy in junior basketball players: a controlled clinical and ultrasonographic study of 268 patellar tendons in players aged 14–18 years. Scand J Med Sci Sports 10(4):216–220
14. Lian Ø, Refsnes PE, Engebretsen L, Bahr R (2003) Performance characteristics of volleyball players with patellar tendinopathy. Am J Sports Med 31(3):408–413
15. Khan KM, Cook JL, Bonar F, Harcourt P, Astrom M (1999) Histopathology of common tendinopathies. Update and implications for clinical management. Sports Med 27(6):393–408
16. Rauh M, Parker R (2009) Patellar and quadriceps tendinopathiesand ruptures. In: DeLee JC (ed) DeLee and Drez's orthopaedic sports medicine. Saunders, Philadelphia, pp 192–200
17. Zernicke RF, Garhammer J, Jobe FW (1977) Human patellar-tendon rupture. J Bone Joint Surg Am 59(2):179–183
18. Magra M, Maffulli N (2008) Genetic aspects of tendinopathy. J Sci Med Sport 24:167–173
19. Magra M, Maffulli N (2005) Matrix metalloproteases: a role in overusetendinopathies. Br J Sports Med 39:789–791
20. Lee D, Stinner D, Mir H (2013) Quadriceps and patellar tendon ruptures. J Knee Surg 26:301–308
21. Herzog W (2000) Muscle properties and coordination during voluntary movement. J Sports Sci 18(3):141–152
22. McNitt-Gray JL (2000) Musculoskeletal loading during landing. In: Biomechanics in sport, vol 9, Encyclopaedia of sports medicine. Blackwell Science, Oxford
23. Sharma P, Maffulli N (2005) Tendon Injury and tendinopathy: healing and repair. J Bone Joint Surg Am 87:187–202
24. Cook JL, Khan KM, Harcourt PR, Grant M, Young DA, Bonar SF (1997) A cross sectional study of 100 athletes with jumper's knee managed conservatively and surgically. The Victorian Institute of Sport Tendon Study Group. Br J Sports Med 31(4):332–336
25. Khan KM, Bonar F, Desmond PM, Cook JL, Young DA, Visentini PJ, Fehrmann MW, Kiss ZS, O'Brien PA, Harcourt PR, Dowling RJ, O'Sullivan RM, Crichton KJ, Tress BM, Wark JD (1996) Patellar tendinosis (jumper's knee): findings at histopathologic examination, US, and MR imaging. Victorian Institute of Sport Tendon Study Group. Radiology 200(3):821–827
26. Lian Ø, Scott A, Engebretsen L, Bahr R, Duronio V, Khan K (2007) Excessive apoptosis in patellar tendinopathy in athletes. Am J Sports Med 35(4):605–611, Epub 2007 Jan 23
27. Karantanas AH, Zibis AH, Papanikolaou N (2001) Increased signal intensity on fat-suppressed three-dimensional T1-weighted pulse sequences in patellar tendon: magic angle effect? Skeletal Radiol 30(2):67–71
28. Yu JS, Popp JE, Kaeding CC, Lucas J (1995) Correlation of MR imaging and pathologic findings in athletes undergoing surgery for chronic patellar tendinitis. AJR Am J Roentgenol 165(1):115–118
29. El-Khoury GY, Wira RL, Berbaum KS, Pope TL Jr, Monu JU (1992) MR imaging of patellar tendinitis. Radiology 184(3):849–854
30. Magra M, Maffulli N (2006) Nonsteroidal anti-inflammatory drugs in tendinopathy. Clin J Sport Med 16:1–3
31. De Girolamo L, Stanco D, Galliera E, Viganò M, Lovati AB, Marazzi MG, Romeo P, Sansone V (2014) Soft-focused extracorporeal shock waves increase the expression of tendon-specific markers and the release of anti-inflammatory cytokines in an adherent culture model of primary human tendon cells. Ultrasound Med Biol 40(6):1

32. Furia JP, Rompe JD, Cacchio A, Del Buono A, Maffulli N (2013) A single application of low-energy radial extracorporeal shock wave therapy is effective for the management of chronic patellar tendinopathy. Knee Surg Sports Traumatol Arthrosc 21(2):346–350
33. Volpi P, Quaglia A, Schoenhuber H, Melegati G, Corsi MM, Banfi G, de Girolamo L (2010) Growth factors in the management of sport-induced tendinopathies: results after 24 months from treatment. A pilot study. J Sports Med Phys Fitness 50(4):494–500
34. Smith J, Sellon JL (2014) Comparing PRP injections with ESWT for athletes with chronic patellar tendinopathy. Clin J Sport Med 24(1):88–89
35. Moraes VY, Lenza M, Tamaoki MJ, Faloppa F, Belloti JC (2014) Platelet-rich therapies for musculoskeletal soft tissue injuries. Cochrane Database Syst Rev 4, CD010071
36. Fukashiro S, Komi PV, Jarvinen M et al (1995) In vivo Achilles tendon loading during jumping in humans. Eur J Appl Physiol Occup Physiol 5:453–458
37. Rees JD, Lichtwark GA, Wolman RL, Wilson AM (2008) The mechanism for efficacy of eccentric loading in Achilles tendon injury; an in vivo study in humans. Rheumatology 47:1493–1497
38. Dejour H, Denjean S, Neyret P (1992) Treatment of old or recurrent ruptures of the patellar ligament by contralateral autograft. Rev Chir Orthop Reparatrice Appar Mot 78(1):58–62

Chapter 12
Hindfoot Tendinopathies

Francesco Allegra, Enrico Bonacci, and Francesco Martinelli

Abstract Posttraumatic tendon disorders and their sequelae involve ankle joint and hindfoot in sport and work-related activities much more than other districts. Ankle trauma represented incidence is 37 sprains every 1000 persons, with an increase in progressive tendency. The ankle is the most involved joint in traumatic pathology and represents 10–15 % of all sports injuries. The pathology of the anterior compartment is most prevalent with a progressive involvement of the posterior compartment of no less importance. Numerous risk factors can contribute in hindfoot and posterior ankle disorders development, intrinsic patient related to its physical form and activities, extrinsic equipment, and environmental conditions related to where the activity is practiced. The population with less than 25 years is the most involved in working and sporting activities with the fibular ligament and posterior tendon compartment involvement. Better coordination between muscle and training activities addressed to the perception of balance makes possible to prevent trauma, resulting in improved muscle strength and improved proprioceptive response from the ankle. Conservative treatment is the first one and represents the 85 % of recoveries. About 15 % needs a surgical treatment, performed preferably by arthroscopic procedure.

12.1 Background

Hindfoot is an anatomic district placed in the posterior ankle and lengthened along the superior aspect of calcaneal tuberosity. It is not an articular space, but two joints are posteriorly opened on this, the ankle joint and the subtalar one. Hindfoot can be subdivided into three parts. The first one is anterior in direct relationship with the

F. Allegra (✉) • E. Bonacci • F. Martinelli
Ortopedia Universitaria, Università La Sapienza,
Polo Pontino, c/o I.C.O.T., Via Francesco Faggiana 1668, Latina 00040, Italy
e-mail: francescoallegra@tin.it; bonacci822@gmail.com; francesco.martinelli@aol.it

G.N. Bisciotti, P. Volpi (eds.), *The Lower Limb Tendinopathies*,
Sports and Traumatology, DOI 10.1007/978-3-319-33234-5_12

two joints and with the posterior tendons of the calf, both medial and lateral. The second one is the widest on sagittal plane and is represented by the cortical bone of upper calcaneal tuberosity. The third one is limited to the last part of Achilles' tendon and its insertion. The presence of many tendinous structures placed both on medial and lateral of posterior ankle side characterizes the district and its typical pathologies. Most of those has a traumatic or micro-traumatic etiology due to musculoskeletal injuries of the lower limb. When patients present with foot and ankle pain, tendinopathies are often missed and assumed to be evaluated by the family doctor just as an ankle sprain, which can lead to chronic pain. The overuse tendon injuries are the most difficult to diagnose because of the slow progression of the disease and the poorness of symptoms from its beginning. Because the tendinopathies have often evolved in a period of years, the tendon condition is considered a degenerative process, affecting the approach to treatment which varies depending on the stage and the etiology of the disorder.

12.2 Biomechanics and Pathophysiology

The biomechanics is fundamental understanding of the patho-mechanics injury mechanisms. The foot and ankle vary its position on the ground following the gait cycle, from the point of initial contact with the ground and heel strike to the point at which the same foot hits the ground again. This cycle is divided into the stance phase (60 %) when the foot is in direct contact with the ground and the swing phase (40 %) when the foot is not in contact with the ground. At heel strike, the foot is supinated, changing immediately after when the foot begins to pronate, becoming maximally pronated at mid-distance. This pronation is normal as the subtalar joint unlocks so the foot can become flexible, while calcaneal tuberosity is in full contact with the ground allowing for accommodation to its surface. As the body weight shifts forward, the foot begins to return to a neutral position in preparation for incoming heel lift. This occurs at the end of the stance phase when the foot starts to supinate, thanks to the resulting in the formation of a rigid subtalar joint which makes easy, valid, and strong toe off. Every abnormality in this simple gait cycle can develop the risk of tendinopathies, especially in the hindfoot. The word tendinopathy is widely used for overuse tendon injuries describing a spectrum of several diagnoses involving injury to the tendon like tendinitis, peritendinitis, and tendinosis, in the absence of one secure pathological diagnosis [1–3]. These overuse disorders are commonly considered to occur when intensity, duration, and mode of specific physical activity, work, or sport training changes in some way. In the absence of such conditions, also the presence of not completely recovered posterior ankle bony fractures, the presence of ankle ligaments insufficiency and the appearance of initial joint arthritis as consequence of former traumas can induce the development of tendinopathies. Generally a period of recovery and rest is sufficient to reduce the increased demands on the tissues, worsening any symptom in case of inadequate recovery, because it influences the breakdown at the cellular level [4]. When the tendon is injured, normal response consists of inflammation followed by deposition of collagen matrix within the tendon, accompanied by a weak remodeling response [1]. However, a failed healing response may occur because of ongoing mechanical forces on the tendon, frequently in association with poor blood supply because of both strangulation of small vessels and weak capability of new local angiogenesis. The continuing such mechanical stimulation produces microscopic tendon structure changes, including fibrin deposition, neovascularization, reduction in white blood cells and macrophages, and finally an increase in collagen breakdown and synthesis, consisting of a disorganized matrix tissue with the presence of hypercellularity and hypervascularity. This tissue has the characteristic to be painful and weak [5, 6].

12.3 Clinical Examination

A history of trauma, involvement in a new sport or exercise, or an increase in the intensity of basic physical activity is always present. Checking the biomechanical alignment of the foot and ankle while the patient is standing and throughout the gait cycle represents a fundamental for pointing tendons disorder out. Understanding the relationship between the different bones of the hindfoot is essential for a correct diagnosis of tendinopathies. Hindfoot tendon dysfunction characteristically is a slow onset condition mainly affecting middle-aged, obese women, even the sporters can be affected with. At the patient's visit, the first foot examination must exclude any calcaneal deformity, acquired or congenital. Degenerative changes in hindfoot medial tendons lead to pain and weakness, progressing to deformity of the foot, and degenerative changes in the surrounding joints. Patients will complain of medial foot pain and weakness and can slowly develop a progressive flatfoot deformity, which is always announced and accompanied with continuous local pain, swelling, and difficulties in walking. Patients affected with hindfoot tendinopathy present seldom an insidious onset of pain over the affected tendon which worsens with sustained activity. In the early stages of disease, pain decreases with a warm-up period; on opposite in later stages, pain may be present at rest but worsens with activity [7]. The pain is less severe during prolonged rest periods. Pain is usually described as far and dull at nighttime rest and as sharp as the activity increases during the day life. No systemic symptoms should be present. Observing the affected area, asymmetry, swelling, or muscle atrophy is checked. Palpation may reveal tenderness along the tendon, reproducing the patient's pain and decreasing range of motion of the affected side. Pain in multiple tendons or joints may represent a rheumatologic cause. Risk factors include obesity, hypertension, diabetes, steroid use, and seronegative arthropathies.

12.4 Instrumental Diagnosis

Plain radiography is recommended as the initial imaging study. X-ray plain weight-bearing anteroposterior and lateral scan of both feet, in addition to bilateral weight-bearing ankle views, should be suggested for a first evaluation of the patient.

Changes may not be apparent on X-ray in the early stages, but as the disease progresses, collapse of the medial longitudinal arch and joint degeneration may become sometimes evident [8]. Results are usually normal, but the study may reveal osteoarthritis, loose body, or a calcification of the tendon. Ultrasound is a quick, readily available, low-cost investigation which gives information about the tendon size, degeneration, and presence of fluid. It is useful for obtaining a dynamic examination and should be compared with tendons on the other side to make certain there is no pathological change. In the tendinosis, tendon is thickened, more or less fusiform, and hypoechoic. Gradually, microlesions appear as longitudinal fissures, and finally the tendon wears thin and loses its normal mechanical properties although its continuity seems to be at least partially maintained. In the tenosynovitis suffusion of the sheath, thickening and hyperemia of the synovia on Doppler are variably associated, possibly occurring before, during, or after a rupture. Some segments of the hindfoot tendons are in close proximity to the ankle ligaments and retinacula, and this is probably a source of error, which can be corrected. However the quality of results can be ultrasonographer dependent [9].

Magnetic resonance imaging (MRI) also provides good images of tendon pathology, especially if surgical evaluation is being considered. There is a significant association with regard to the presence of tendon abnormalities (tendinosis, tenosynovitis, and tearing) in both the peroneal and medial flexor tendons [10]. The complex interconnected system of retaining fascia and retinacula in the distal aspect of the leg, just above and at the level of the ankle, creates distinct tendon compartments. Furthermore, recent evidence has shown that these and other retinacula also play a functional role, as they are not simply static structures for joint stabilization, like ligaments, but rather provide local spatial proprioception during movements of the foot and ankle [11]. A statistical correlation was found between the diameters and sectional areas of most of the ankle and hindfoot tendons, as well as between qualitative abnormalities on MR images of these tendons. This association seems to indicate that abnormalities in one of the tendons may influence the integrity of the other tendons perhaps on the basis of a retinacular and fascial system that connects them [11]. Regarding the posterior tibial tendon dysfunction alone, some authors relieved a confirmation to the statistically significant link between posterior tibial tendon and injuries found on the MRI in key structures for the stabilization of plantar arch, like the spring ligament and tarsal sinus ligaments. Similarly they found a high statistically significant frequency of calcaneal spur and talus peaks in patients affected with same district dysfunction [12].

12.5 Treatment

As considered before, hindfoot tendon injuries are not inflammatory in nature. Medical treatment should be limited to use nonsteroidal anti-inflammatory drugs (NSAIDs) alone to provide short-term pain relief for patients with tendinopathy but do not affect long-term outcomes. Treatment of such disorders ranges from relative rest to surgical debridement. However, many therapies have not been studied in clinical trials, and it is not known whether the same treatment options can be applied to all tendinopathies. The conservative measures are considered the "golden standard" including protection, relative rest, ice, compression, elevation, local medications, and rehabilitative exercise modalities. At the beginning, patients should be encouraged to reduce their level of physical activity with the immediate aim to reduce and stop repetitive loading on the tendon depending on the injury and the day life activity and the timing of relative rest [13]. Furthermore, any therapy must begin by the medical evaluation of both the extrinsic and intrinsic causes of tendon injury. Extrinsic factors include overuse of the tendon, training errors, smoking, medication abuse, and wearing shoes or other equipments not appropriate for the specific patient's activity. The use of unappropriated type of shoes for the patient's foot type such as motion control, cushioned, or stability must be discouraged . Flexibility and strength of the tendon, patient age, leg length, and vascular supply may also play a role evaluated as intrinsic factors. Although identifying and treating these factors have been the mainstay of treatment over the years, evidence on their effectiveness is lacking [3]. Orthotics, such as inserts or a heel wedge, are sometimes used to help unload, reinforce, and protect the tendon. Eccentric strength training, which involves actively lengthening the muscle, is an effective therapy that helps promote the formation of new collagen. Eccentric exercise has proved beneficial in the treatment of Achilles and patellar tendinosis, and it may be helpful in other tendinopathies as well [5]. Other physical therapy modalities include ultrasound, iontophoresis (electric charge to drive medication into the tissues), and phonophoresis (the use of ultrasound to enhance the delivery of topically applied drugs), but little evidence exists on their effectiveness in treating tendinopathy. Because many of the standard therapies for tendinopathy have failed in time to correct and stop the tendon degenerative process, many new treatments are being developed. These include extracorporeal shock wave therapy [14], radiofrequency ablation, percutaneous tenotomy, autologous blood, or growth factor injection; the effectiveness of these treatments are being currently investigated.

If a comprehensive, custom-made, nonsurgical treatment program of 3–6 months has failed, surgery should be considered only if the patient is unwilling to alter his or her level of physical activity or if rupture of the tendon is evident. The final aim of each surgical treatment is the excision of the tendon release of impinging bony or soft tissue including abnormal scarring and fibrosis tissue.

12.6 Single Site Tendinopathies

12.6.1 Tibialis Posterior Tendon

The function of posterior tibial tendon is to flex plantarly the foot and to activate the inversion of the foot, stabilizing the medial longitudinal arch in the same time. Posterior tibialis tendinopathy is a prevalent musculoskeletal condition often resulting in gait abnormalities along with medial ankle and foot pain. The disorders of this tendon can lead to a painful flatfoot deformity with the consequence of overstress to the midfoot ligaments in the calcaneonavicular joint and to deltoid ligament, whose elongation can worsen the medial ankle instability in association with flatfoot.

As predisposing condition for posterior tibial tendinopathy is gender, female much more than male and 40 years aged at mean, without previous acute trauma, present in patient's clinical report. The history of a far previous traumatic event to the ankle joint, often misdiagnosed as involving the medial compartment, can be considered the cause of posterior tibial tendon synovitis in the majority of these patients. Symptoms can be referred to a sudden unexpected loss of balance because of slipping of curb or slipping on a stair or stepping in a hole, recovered in a short time but remained painful and dull in any activity. Morphology and vascularization of painful tibialis posterior should be examined, targeting the degenerated tendon. The symptomatic foot can be deformed in an excessive pronation due to the weakness of the posterior tibial muscle and tendon compared with the other side: it is especially evident when patient is requested to maintain a tiptoe standing or walking. When symptoms occur the patient is no more able to single leg and toe raise, associated with the impossibility to have an active and strong plantar flexion of the involved foot. The presence of swelling and foot deformity because of posterior tibial tendinopathy gradually increases in irregular but continuous way, by months to years, progressing symptoms in the opposite side of the ankle joint in the region of sinus tarsi below the fibular malleolus.

Treatment is at beginning conservative and must be initiated promptly because of the risk of progressive deterioration and a nonfunctional tendon. Non-operative treatment can alleviate symptoms and control progression in nearly all stages of the disease. Immobilization in a leg cast or cast boot is suggested for a period of some weeks depending on the symptom recovery. Local injection of hyaluronate can be considered an option because of the effect on inflamed tendon and sheath; furthermore, the use of steroids into synovia are discouraged because of the high rate of tendon rupture secondary to local necrotic effect on tenocytes. Physiotherapy and rehabilitation are considered a valid option. The posterior tibialis muscle is able to perform efficiently at the initial stage by restoring cuboid internal rotation mobility, associated with midtarsal pronation and lower extremity neuromuscular control: activating this rehabilitation in time resolves the chronic tendinopathy and permits the patient to optimum functional ability returning [15]. Despite strengthening and stretching exercises combined with orthosis treatment in a home-based program, which has been evaluated as valid conservative treatment, a moderate-intensity, home-based exercise program is evaluated as minimally effective, in augmenting orthosis wear alone in patients with tibialis posterior tendinopathy disorder stage II [16]. In examining the degenerated tendon by grayscale imaging and Doppler ultrasound at initial and posttreatment stage, to assess the tendon's morphology and signs of neovascularization with functional status and patient pain level, a program of rehabilitation can be lead out: a 10-week tendon-specific eccentric program resulted in improvements in symptoms and function without changes in tendon morphology or neovascularization [17].

If conservative management fails for up to 3 months or if stage 3 flatfoot deformities are diagnosed, the patient should be referred to an orthopedic surgeon. Insufficiency or rupture of the posterior tibial tendon is a frequent cause of adult acquired flatfoot deformity, considered as a common clinical disorder. Its early recognition is essential because natural history is characterized by progressively worsening deformity. Surgical solution should be considered at failure of symptom control or at prevention of deformity progression. In early stage 1, an arthroscopic surgical procedure should be indicated to explore the tendon and its sheath along (Fig. 12.1), following this structure behind the tibial malleolus: a debridement of the inflamed tissue of synovia or a removal of symptomatic partial tendon tear (see Fig. 12.2) should be performed using two small medial side portal. In stage 1,

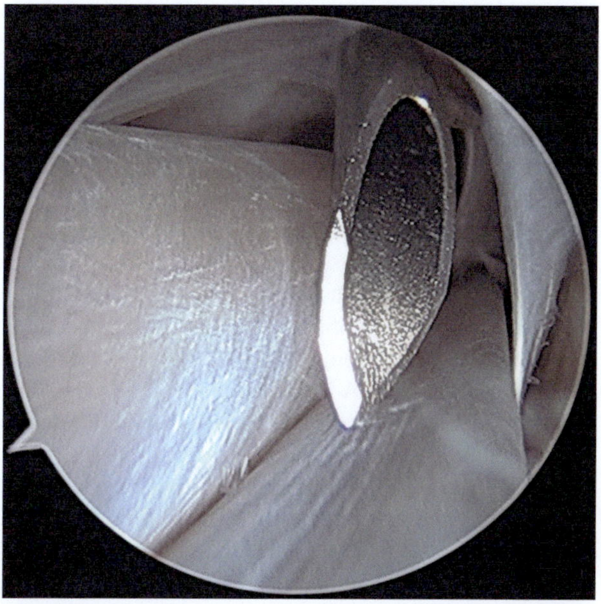

Fig. 12.1 In this arthroscopic image, the posterior tibialis tendon lies below the spinal needle tip, used as a probe in the restricted space of the tendon sheath

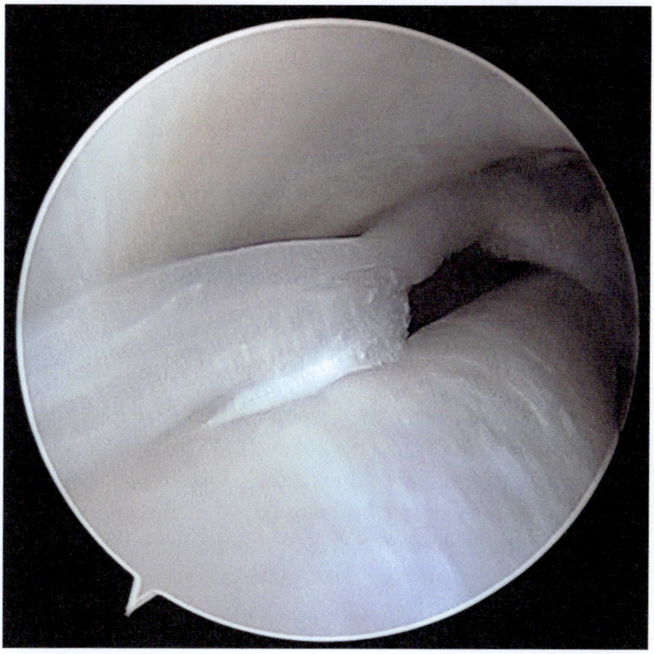

Fig. 12.2 The arthroscopic visualization allows the surgeon to finalize the diagnosis, finding a partial rupture of posterior tibialis tendon easy to be remodeled by shaver introduced in a proximal portal

exploration and debridement with or without flexor digitorum longus (FDL) tendon transfer is a surgical option. In stage 2, the tendon becomes elongated involving a reduction of medial soft tissues. Exploration and debridement of the PTT is performed, but frequently a FDL tendon transfer or side-to-side anastomosis is required performing with an open procedure. In the stage 2b, the treatment addressed on soft tissue alone may fail to resolve patient's symptoms: correct bony deformity should be considered in this stage a valid option to avoid deterioration of results over time even surgery limited only to tendon. Combined procedures, including soft tissue reconstructions to restore PTT function and bony procedures to correct deformity, are considered more safe and durable at outcome. In stage I or early stage II, when the posterior tibial tendon appears intact with minimal degeneration or elongation, a further surgical step to reconstruct the medial column may be considered: an advancement of osteoperiosteal flap based on the tendon insertion is suggested to be combined with selective bony medial column arthrodesis. Although it may be theoretically possible to passively correct hindfoot valgus with these procedures, it seems prudent to limit the indications to patients who have early disease accompanied by an isolated midfoot sag. In more advanced stage II disease, correction of deformity with a tendon transfer alone is incorrect because it is not sufficient to repair the deformity. A combined open procedure addressed to the bone with a medial displacement calcaneal osteotomy or a lateral column lengthening is currently recommended, correcting the deformity and sparing of the hindfoot joints: its advantage is particularly evident in young or active patients. In stage 3, arthrodesis is the procedure of choice because the deformity is fixed and the joints appear to be stiff: the procedure changes depending on the joints affected and the columns of ankle and foot involved. Long-standing results are present when the deformity is approached with isolated talonavicular arthrodesis, correcting all its clinical and radiological aspects; however, in recovering the hindfoot from a complete loss of motion, the appearance of closer joint arthritis is the price to be paid. This clinical situation is not rare, and in a large number of patients, the triple arthrodesis is probably preferred. If residual deformity or instability is present after these procedures, it must be treated. Residual medial column instability may be addressed by adding a selective arthrodesis of the naviculo-cuneiform or first metatarso-cuneiform joint, whereas residual forefoot varus or supination may be addressed with selected midfoot fusions with or without a cuneiform osteotomy.

12.6.2 Peroneal Tendons

Chronic tendinitis, tendinosis, and interstitial tears are more common disorders of peroneal tendon, but complete tear and subluxation at posterior edge of fibular malleolus are also frequent. Often due to ankle joint injury, they are a consequence of lateral ankle instability and are the main cause of the lateral symptoms of the joint [18]. Injuries can be acute as a result of trauma or present as chronic problems, often in patients with predisposing structural components such as hindfoot varus, lateral ligamentous instability, an enlarged peroneal tubercle, and a symptomatic os peroneum. Because it is a common subjective feeling of ankle giving way, often without sure symptoms of instability, it is very important that the patient should be submitted to a visit of a specialist to evaluate the possibility to stabilize the joint [19]. Persistent lateral ankle swelling, popping, and retro-fibular pain often occurring are typical symptoms of tendinitis. Tendon subluxation is a common disorder characterized by popping and giving way sensation: a positive peroneal tunnel compression test is painful, with active dorsiflexion and eversion of the foot against resistance along the posterior ridge of the fibula. The evidence of subluxation and/or dislocation of the peroneal tendons should be referred to an orthopedist [18]. Also rheumatoid arthritis or a seronegative arthropathy is considered as a cause of symptoms as swelling and tenderness, especially in the absence of increased work or sport activity or trauma. It is generally difficult to refer patient's clinical findings for peroneal pathology and magnetic resonance imaging (MRI), utilized for diagnosing peroneal tendon pathology. However, patients with MRI findings of peroneal tendon pathology should undergo careful clinical examination, as the positive predictive value of MRI for peroneal tendon pathology with actual clinical findings is low [20]. On the other hand, studies demonstrate that peroneal tendon tears are often incidental findings on MRI [21]. Patients with chronic lateral ankle instability also have peroneal tendinopathy often. However, preoperative MRIs of patients affected with peroneal tendon tendinopathy are vague in many cases, especially in those with chronic lateral ankle instability, despite that it is a useful diagnostic tool for detecting such peroneal disorders. Therefore, a thorough delicate physical examination and careful observation is always needed [22].

Conservative treatment is the first to be prescribed to patients. Lateral heel wedges and ankle taping help unload stress on the peroneal tendon, but there is no evidence that they induce healing. Rehabilitation therapy involves ankle range-of-motion exercises, peroneal strengthening, proper warm-up, and proprioception activity. Indications for surgery include failure of conservative management, recurrent peroneal instability, and rupture of the peroneal tendon. Any instable ankle should be stabilized on the surgeon's indication, reconstructing ligaments, or performing surgical procedure to fix injured ligaments or joint stabilizing structures. Also subluxation and/or dislocation of the peroneal tendons should be submitted to an orthopedic surgeon to evaluate the opportunity to reconstruct the posterior fibular retinacula or to treat with a different surgical procedure to stabilize tendons in their own bony groove. Arthroscopic surgery has a reserved space for those peroneal tendons disorders (see Fig. 12.3) limited to symptomatic tendinitis and tendinosis (see Fig. 12.4) or to partial ruptures secondary to posterior ankle soft tissue or bony impingement.

12.6.3 Flexor Hallucis Longus Tendon

Tendinopathy of the flexor hallucis longus (FHL), colloquially referred to as "dancer's tendinitis," is a common condition in dancers and attributed to high demand on this muscle in positions of extreme ankle plantarflexion and

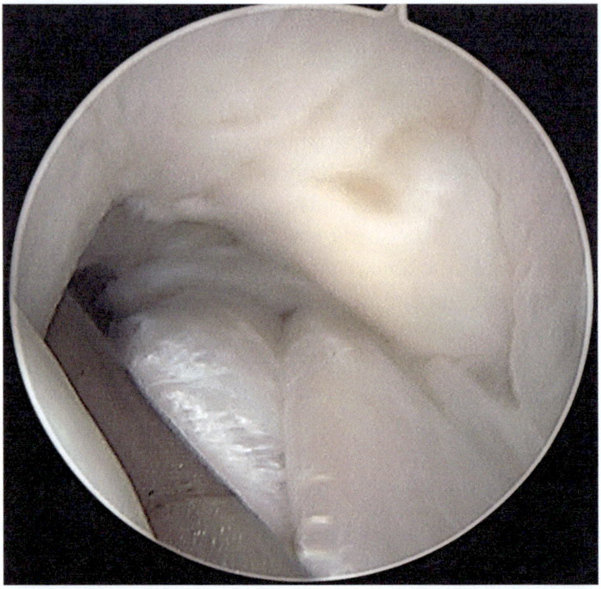

Fig. 12.3 The peroneal tendons appear inside their sheath; place the peroneal brevis close to probe instrument and the peroneal longus closer to internal aspect of peroneal malleolus. The movement of the probe permits an exploration of the tendons under direct visualization of the scope

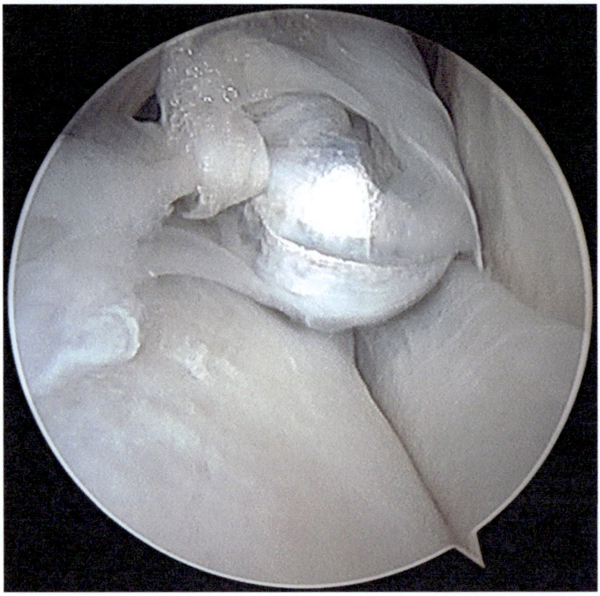

Fig. 12.4 The shaver is approaching to the scope from an anterior and lower portal and is going to debride tendons from the symptomatic synovial tissue

metatarsophalangeal (MTP) flexion and extension. Despite that this injury is the most common lower extremity tendinitis in classical ballet dancers [23], it is also seen in persons who participate in activities requiring frequent push-off maneuvers [24]. Tenosynovitis of the flexor hallucis longus (FHL) tendon is a condition typically found in some sports like in soccer players, related to chronic overuse.

A traumatic cause for this situation, such as an ankle sprain, is considered rare. This particular kind of tendinitis of the hindfoot is almost always caused by the FHL entrapment, like it is realized in the "en pointe" position of dancers, leading to a chronic pain, early arthritis, and fibrosis with progressive decreased range of motion. At the beginning, the onset of symptoms is along the posteromedial aspect of the ankle behind the malleolus or less frequently on the medial side of subtalar joint below the tip of medial malleolus. During the visit, when the doctor asks the patient to plantar flex the great toe against the resistance or to stand and to walk on tiptoe, the pain suddenly appears with an occasional crepitus along the posterior edge of tibial malleolus. A useful clinical test is to compare the passive extension of the first metatarsophalangeal joint with the foot and ankle in the neutral and plantar flexed assessment: when a little or no extension in neutral position is checked, disappearing in plantar flexion, the FHL tendon appears to be entrapped.

Prevention includes reducing turnout of the hip to make the dancer working directly over the foot and avoiding hard floors whenever possible. Strengthening the body's core is one of the main rehabilitation activities to balance strength and to develop the muscles which stabilize and move the trunk of the body such as abdominal, back, and pelvic muscles. The use of firm and well-fitted shoes can be considered a good prevention; however, less possible in dancers whose relatively stiff feet may contribute to the disorder because of the incorrect en pointe position. For the athlete who is specialized in sprint sports (run, soccer, football), it is important to wear appropriate shoes and to correct the starting moment, to avoid overcharging the tendon. For prolonged tendinitis, 2–3 weeks of immobilization in a weight-bearing cast or walking boot is recommended. Efficacy of using modified heel raise task with the toes off the edge of a block as a means to train larger plantarflexors is proposed as therapy and as prevention. Improving interventions for FHL tendinopathy will be impactful for dancers, in whom this condition is highly prevalent and be considered valid for all the workers which are frequently submitted to.

In case of failure of conservative treatment, the tendon can be surgically released, which is usually done through an open procedure. But by years it has been validated also that the arthroscopic procedure, which can release the FHL with a very low surgical aggression, allowed good visualization of the involved structures and yielded good results. This condition can be related to multiple microtraumas, not remaining an exclusive disease of ballet dancers or overuse [25]. Open and arthroscopic techniques have been utilized in the treatment of posterior impingement of the ankle and hindfoot. Because posterior impingement occurs more frequently in patients who repetitively plantarflex the ankle, this population may especially benefit from a procedure that reduces pain and results in maximal range of motion (ROM). Posterior ankle endoscopy allowed for maintenance or restoration of anatomic ROM of the ankle and hindfoot, ability to return to at least previous level of activity, and improvement in objective assessment of pain relief and higher level of function parameters. Complications associated with this procedure were minimal [26]. Hindfoot endoscopic surgery has been described as a minimally

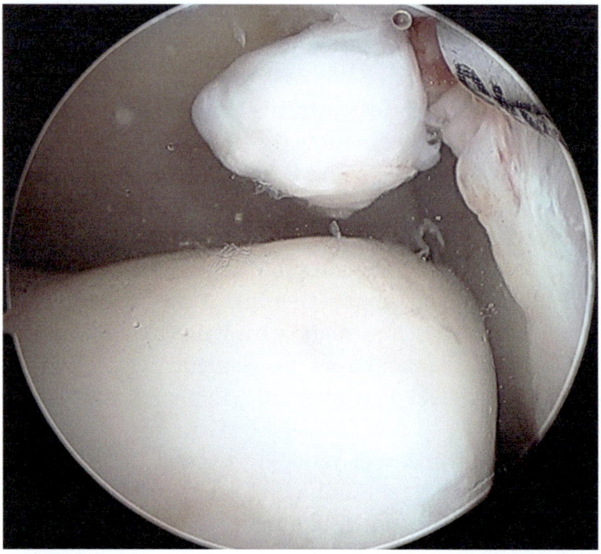

Fig. 12.5 The presence of a cartilaginous loose body can be occasionally cause of hindfoot tendon impingement: its removal releases completely the disorders

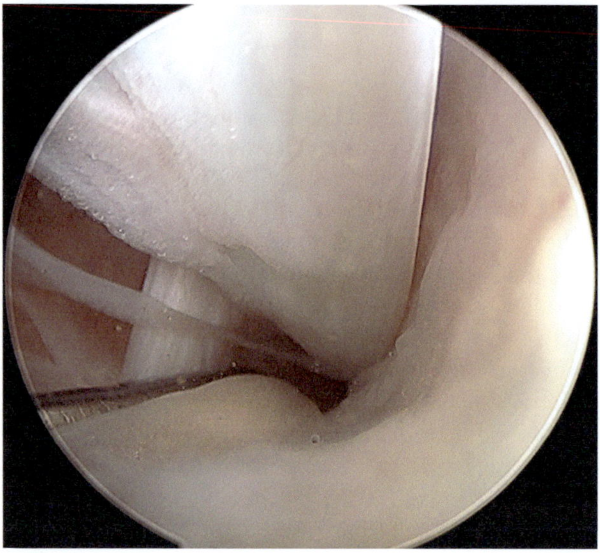

Fig. 12.6 The FHL tendon can also impinge inside its sheath behind the posterior edge of tibial malleolus, where its path curves to become straight, passing into the foot plant

invasive surgical treatment for posterior ankle and FHL impingement syndrome [27] removing the possible causes of impingement as posterior loose body (Fig. 12.5) or removing fibrous tissue from the sheath at its hindfoot origin (Fig. 12.6) until complete tendon release (Fig. 12.7). With this procedure, a systematic approach for identifying relevant hindfoot structures and its abnormalities during hindfoot

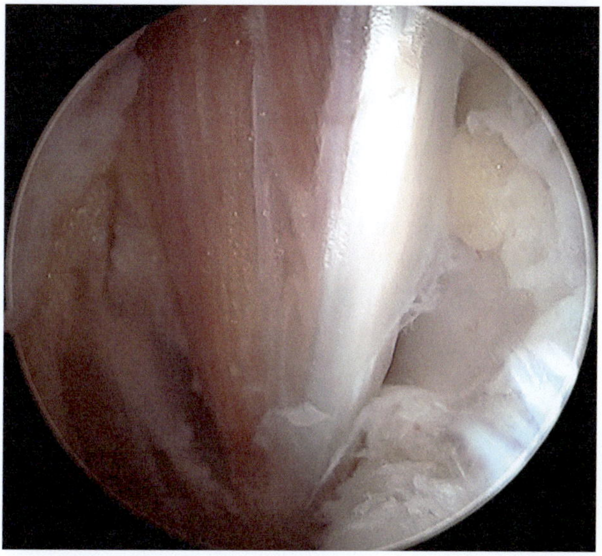

Fig. 12.7 The FHL tendon is completely released and it moves up and down, following the passive movements the surgeon impresses the great toe

exploration is possible, dividing the extra-articular structures of the hindfoot into quadrants as defined by the intermalleolar ligament. Hindfoot arthroscopic surgery is an effective treatment strategy for posterior ankle FHL impingement syndrome [28]. In addition, it allows the patients a rapid return to sporting activities.

12.7 Conclusions

Hindfoot tendinopathies are less frequent and dependent on the patient's activity. Despite the absence of data, possible risk factors have been assumed such as age, duration of symptoms, body mass index, type of tendinopathy, previous therapies, and the presence of associated ankle injuries. At their appearance the right and fast diagnosis leads to the correct treatment, in time to avoid symptoms to become chronic. Patients must be firstly submitted to conservative therapy, remaining the specific indication for surgery only at failure of any other treatments. Advances in foot and ankle arthroscopy have allowed surgeons to diagnose and treat a broadening array of disorders that were previously limited to open procedures. Arthroscopy of the posterior ankle, hindfoot, and tendoscopy can be used to address common ankle ailments, with the potential benefits of decreased pain, fast recovery, and low complication rates. Posterior ankle arthroscopy can be indicated to manage impingement, arthrofibrosis, and synovitis which are the most common causes of hindfoot tendinopathies. Tendoscopy is a minimally invasive alternative for evaluation and debridement of the posterior tibial, flexor hallucis longus, and peroneal tendons.

References

1. Maffulli N, Khan KM, Puddu G (1998) Overuse tendon conditions: time to change a confusing terminology. Arthroscopy 14(8):840–843
2. Wilder RP, Sethi S (2004) Overuse injuries: tendinopathies, stress fractures, compartment syndrome, and shin splints. Clin Sports Med 23(1):55–81
3. Plattner PF (1989) Tendon problems of the foot and ankle. The spectrum from peritendinitis to rupture. Postgrad Med 86(3):155–170
4. O'Connor FG, Nirschl RP, Howard TM (1997) Managing overuse injuries. Phys Sportsmed 25(5):88–113
5. Khan KM, Cook JL, Bonar F, Harcourt P, Astrom M (1999) Histopathology of common tendinopathies. Update and implications for clinical management. Sports Med 27(6):393–408
6. Leadbetter WB (1992) Cell-matrix response in tendon injury. Clin Sports Med 11(3):533–578
7. Bubra PS, Keighley GS, Rateesh S, Carmody D (2015) Posterior tibial tendon dysfunction: an overlooked cause of foot deformity. J Family Med Prim Care 4:26–29
8. Pedowitz WJ, Kovatis P (1995) Flatfoot in the adult. J Am Acad Orthop Surg 3:293–302
9. Lhoste-Trouilloud A (2012) The tibialis posterior tendon. J Ultrasound 15:2–6
10. Stecco C, Macchi V, Porzionato A et al (2010) The ankle retinacula: morphological evidence of the proprioceptive role of the fascial system. Cells Tissues Organs 192(3):200–210
11. Cabral P, Paulino C, Takahashi R, Clopton P, Resnick D (2013) Correlation of morphologic and pathologic features of the various tendon groups around the ankle: MR imaging investigation. Skeletal Radiol 42:1393–1402
12. Herráiz Hidalgo L, Carrascoso Arranz J, Recio Rodríguez M, Jiménez de la Peña M, Cano Alonso R, Álvarez Moreno E, Martínez de Vega Fernández V (2014) Posterior tibial tendon dysfunction: what other structures are involved in the development of acquired adult flat foot? Radiologia 56(3):247–256
13. Jones DC (1993) Tendon disorders of the foot and ankle. J Am Acad Orthop Surg 1(2):87–94
14. Rompe JD, Nafe B, Furia JP, Maffulli N (2007) Eccentric loading, shock-wave treatment, or a wait-and-see policy for tendinopathy of the main body of tendo Achillis: a randomized controlled trial [published correction appears in Am J Sports Med. 2007;35(7):1216]. Am J Sports Med 35(3):374–383
15. Patla C, Lwin J, Smith L, Chaconas E (2015) Cuboid manipulation and exercise in the management of posterior tibialis tendinopathy: a case report. Int J Sports Phys Ther 10(3):363–370
16. Houck J, Neville C, Tome J, Flemister A (2015) Randomized controlled trial comparing orthosis augmented by either stretching or stretching and strengthening for Stage II Tibialis Posterior Tendon Dysfunction. Foot Ankle Int 36(9):1006–1016
17. Kulig K, Lederhaus ES, Reischl S, Arya S, Bashford G (2009) Effect of eccentric exercise program for early tibialis posterior tendinopathy. Foot Ankle Int 30(9):877–885
18. Sammarco GJ (1994) Peroneal tendon injuries. Orthop Clin North Am 25(1):135–145
19. DiGiovanni BF, Fraga CJ, Cohen BE, Shereff MJ (2000) Associated injuries found in chronic lateral ankle instability. Foot Ankle Int 21(10):809–815
20. Giza E, Mak W, Wong SE, Roper G, Campanelli V, Hunter JC (2013) A clinical and radiological study of peroneal tendon pathology. Foot Ankle Spec 6(6):417–421
21. Schubert R (2013) MRI of peroneal tendinopathies resulting from trauma or overuse. Br J Radiol 86(1021):20110750
22. Park HJ, Cha SD, Kim HS, Chung ST, Park NH, Yoo JH, Park JH, Kim JH, Lee TW, Lee CH, Oh SM (2010) Reliability of MRI findings of peroneal tendinopathy in patients with lateral chronic ankle instability. Clin Orthop Surg 2(4):237–243
23. Hamilton WG, Geppert MJ, Thompson FM (1996) Pain in the posterior aspect of the ankle in dancers. Differential diagnosis and operative treatment. J Bone Joint Surg Am 78(10):1491–1500

24. Cooper ME, Wolin PM (1999) Os trigonum syndrome with flexor hallucis longus tenosynovitis in a professional football referee. Med Sci Sports Exerc 31(7 Suppl):S493–S496
25. Corte-Real NM, Moreira RM, Guerra-Pinto F (2012) Arthroscopic treatment of tenosynovitis of the flexor hallucis longus tendon. Foot Ankle Int 33(12):1108–1112
26. Carreira DS, Vora AM, Hearne KL, Kozy J (2016) Outcome of arthroscopic treatment of posterior impingement of the ankle. J Foot Ankle Int 37(4):394–400
27. Smyth NA, Murawski CD, Levine DS, Kennedy JG (2013) Hindfoot arthroscopic surgery for posterior ankle impingement: a systematic surgical approach and case series. Am J Sports Med 41(8):1869–1876
28. Hsu AR, Gross CE, Lee S, Carreira DS (2014) Extended indications for foot and ankle arthroscopy. J Am Acad Orthop Surg 22(1):10–19

Index

G.N. Bisciotti, P. Volpi (eds.), *The Lower Limb Tendinopathies*,
Sports and Traumatology, DOI 10.1007/978-3-319-33234-5

MIX
Papier aus verantwortungsvollen Quellen
Paper from responsible sources
FSC® C105338

If you have any concerns about our products,
you can contact us on
ProductSafety@springernature.com

In case Publisher is established outside the EU,
the EU authorized representative is:
Springer Nature Customer Service Center GmbH
Europaplatz 3, 69115 Heidelberg, Germany

Printed by Libri Plureos GmbH
in Hamburg, Germany